Psalm 139:1-12

O Lord, thou hast searched me, and known me.
Thou knowest my downsitting and mine uprising;
   thou understandest my thought afar off.
Thou compassest my path and my lying down,
   and art acquainted with all my ways.
For there is not a word in my tongue, but, lo, O Lord,
   thou knowest it altogether.
Thou hast beset me behind and before,
   and laid thine hand upon me.
Such knowledge is too wonderful for me;
   it is high, I cannot attain unto it.

Whither shall I go from thy spirit?
   or whither shall I flee from thy presence?
If I ascend up into heaven, thou art there:
   if I make my bed in hell, behold, thou art there.
If I take the wings of the morning,
   and dwell in the uttermost parts of the sea;
Even there shall thy hand lead me,
   and thy right hand shall hold me.
If I say, Surely the darkness shall cover me;
   even the night shall be light about me.
Yea, the darkness hideth not from thee;
   but the night shineth as the day:
   the darkness and the light are both alike to thee.

A New Way to Care for the Dying

A
Hospice
Handbook

Edited by

Michael P. Hamilton
and
Helen F. Reid

GRAND RAPIDS
WILLIAM B. EERDMANS PUBLISHING COMPANY

Copyright © 1980 by William B. Eerdmans Publishing Company
255 Jefferson Ave., S.E., Grand Rapids, Mich. 49503
Printed in the United States of America

Library of Congress Cataloging in Publication Data
Main entry under title:

A Hospice handbook.

   Bibliography: p. 181.
    1. Terminal care. 2. Terminal care facilities.
I. Hamilton, Michael Pollock, 1927-   II. Reid, Helen F.
R726.8.H67   362.1   79-19518
ISBN 0-8028-1802-1

Contents

Preface

SENATOR EDWARD M. KENNEDY

The hospice concept has moved me deeply. It is a truly humane way of caring for the dying. As a member of the United States Senate for the past sixteen years, I have worked diligently to assure quality health care as a right for all Americans. But there is no way any of us in Congress can assure that the care will be delivered in a humane and compassionate way.

Hospice is part of a movement to humanize the way medical care is given. This movement has focused on the beginning as well as the end of life. Natural childbirth—the participation of both parents in the birth process—and the hospice movement both share the common recognition that the family has an important role to play in the health care system. The family understands needs that are beyond the knowledge of the health professional. The family and patient working in concert with the doctor and the nurse can form the most compassionate plan of care.

The family is the basis and the strength of our society. Our families are strengthened by sharing and participating in the death of a loved one. Our lives revolve around our loved ones. Why should life just before death be any different?

In this excellent book we learn that while meeting our medical needs, hospice can also provide emotional and spiritual support and understanding for those facing death. As Dr. Cicely Saunders has said, hospice helps you "live until you die."

Hospice is a reality and a bright light in our health care system. Hospice provides a type of care that must become a model not just for the dying, but for the whole health delivery system. T.S. Eliot could have been speaking of hospice when he said:

> What we call the beginning is often the end
> And to make an end is to make a beginning.

Introduction

The dying are often lonely, frightened, and in pain. They deserve special care and attention, and this book describes a new, humane way to help them. All of us will die one day, and we need to prepare for that time.

The Hospice for the Dying movement began in England in the late fifties and early sixties with the opening of St. Christopher's Hospice in London. It was primarily the creation of Dr. Cicely Saunders, who recognized that many patients were receiving inadequate care in hospitals and that relatives were having problems in caring for the dying at home. Dr. Saunders saw the need for supporting and counselling the patients and their families before death as well as after death. She inaugurated programs by which patients, knowing their death was inevitable and imminent, could enter the hospice program and receive only symptomatic control. Instead of using heroic technological methods which prolonged the dying process, Dr. Saunders gave only sophisticated and effective pain relief. She provided medical, nursing, and spiritual care for hospice resident patients and also for those who, having someone to look after them, could die comfortably and happily in their homes.

Canon Hamilton is on the staff of the Washington Episcopal Cathedral and has long been involved in concerns of medical ethics and delivery of health care services. His previous edited books include The Charismatic Movement *and* To Avoid Catastrophe: A Study in Future Nuclear Weapons Policy.
Helen F. Reid is a poet and editor living in Washington, D.C.

To meet the wide range of patient and family needs, her program required a large number of specially trained nurses and volunteers. St. Christopher's, the result of her extensive research, training, and dedication, was so successful that there are now over fifty operating hospices in the United Kingdom. A few have been established in the United States, and hundreds of others are in various stages of organization. Many politicians, including Senator Kennedy, the author of the preface to this book, and the former Secretary of Health, Education and Welfare, Joseph Califano, have given their support to the goals of the movement.

Our nation is now evaluating various hospice models and searching for the best means to support them financially. The public has become aware of the possibilities offered by the hospice program, and this book will provide both theoretical and practical advice on how a hospice can operate.

The first section outlines, in vivid and personal terms, the needs of the dying. "A Child Dies" was written by a mother after her child died of heart disease. Dr. Rosenbaum's article shows how a sensitive and competent physician uses his personal and professional skills to minister to the dying.

The section entitled "The Response of the Hospice" describes the English hospice movement. In addition, Dr. Sylvia Lack, the noted medical director of the first operational American hospice, in New Haven, Connecticut, writes about the most common of all the pain syndromes—cancer—and how she treats it.

One of the salient concerns of Dr. Cicely Saunders was the integration of religious help for the patient and family into the services provided by other medical and social work disciplines. A mature and sensitive minister, she found, can be of invaluable help as the patient prepares for his or her death and tries to understand its relation to his or her faith or philosophy of life. The role of the chaplain is to help the patient grow spiritually and to support the family before, during, and after death. Another important aspect of a hospice chaplain's duties is working with individual members of the staff and upholding their morale during their arduous work. Some patients and their families are active church members, and they, of course, call on their own priest, pastor, or rabbi. Others, however, have inactive or no church membership, and the services of the hospice chaplain, or other clergy specially trained and associated with the hospice, are then needed. The sacraments can become practical and powerful vehicles of God's concern for those who suffer. Some patients have no desire to enter into explicit religious conversation or relationships, but they do appreciate a chaplain who is simply a loving person willing to provide humane understanding and friendship. The Rev. Paul S. Dawson writes with wisdom and compassion on this ministry.

The last chapter in this section provides a clinical history of the last days of a patient in the hospice wing of the Royal Victoria Hospital in Montreal.

The final section in the book is perhaps the most useful to those readers who want to learn how to organize a hospice in their community. The differences between what a hospice does and what nursing homes and hospitals do are outlined, and the distinctive qualities of a hospice are clarified. In some cases, given organizational clarity and hospital administrators' understanding and support, it is possible for a hospice to be associated with, or part of, a hospital. Dr. Norman Walter has achieved this in the Kaiser Foundation Hospital in California.

The final two chapters are written by people who have been involved in organizing a hospice. One chapter discusses the training of those who have volunteered to help patients and their families, and the other details certification regulations.

*   *   *   *   *

In closing, the editors wish to express their gratitude to many who have made this book possible. First, we are indebted to The Right Reverend John T. Walker, Bishop of the Episcopal Diocese of Washington and Dean of the Cathedral, and also to Canon Charles A. Perry, Provost of the Cathedral, for upholding the broad concept of the ministry of this Cathedral in the nation, and encouraging the development of this book as part of that responsibility.

The funding came from the Cathedral and also from two outside sources: The Coonley Foundation, Inc. and The Paddock Foundation. Their perspicacity in recognizing the contribution of the hospice movement in relieving the suffering of the dying, and their willingness to invest their funds to publicize it through this book are much appreciated. Our thanks also go to our secretary, Jean Buker, who made a major contribution through her careful work.

If this book helps relatives to understand the process of caring for a dying family member, if it aids communities in establishing local hospices, and if it can help a dying person make the pilgrimage from this life to the next with increased peace of mind and physical comfort, then the editors will be greatly rewarded.

The profits, above production costs, will be given to The Washington Hospice Society, Inc.

MICHAEL P. HAMILTON
HELEN F. REID

PART I

THE NEEDS OF THE DYING

I

Lillian Preston Dies of Cancer

SANDOL STODDARD

Lillian Preston, age twenty-nine. She was the only child of
aging parents, reclusive and impoverished gentlefolk. Married
at twenty-two. At twenty-three, abandoned by her husband.
Unable to find work, left with a baby daughter to care for, she
returned in disgrace to the grudging parental home. Job finally
found as a decorator's assistant in London, a two-year struggle
ensuing, to establish a home for herself and her daughter.
Success at last; and then, on their first holiday together, a
boating accident in which the child is drowned. Six months
later, Lillian Preston's doctor tells her that she has cancer,
and that her uterus must be removed. Her uterus is removed,
and after surgery, she is told that her cancer has metastasized
beyond hope of cure. She is admitted to St. Christopher's Hospice, near London.

Mrs. Preston looks now like a woman in her late forties.
She sits in a pale yellow quilted dressing gown, writing notes,
in the armchair beside her bed, her abdomen swollen as if she
were eight months pregnant. She has long, dark hair, bones
like a racehorse, dark eyes and eyebrows, very white skin drawn

*Sandol Stoddard is the author of ten children's books and has
written on a variety of non-fiction subjects for adults. In writing*
The Hospice Movement, *Ms. Stoddard drew on her experience
as a volunteer in St. Christopher's Hospice, London, and her
work in the Hospice of Marin in Marin County, California.*

taut over her cheekbones, an aura about her that is not quite
a trick of the light—a radiance. Prognosis: two weeks.

We talk of this and that. I clear her tray, help her into
bed. Tomorrow the doctors are going to draw off some of the
fluid, she tells me, and then she expects to be more comfortable. Now? Well, not too bad, really, only she is so heavy with
it, and rather sleepy. Strange to feel so peaceful, so secure
now and almost to feel—well, happy, really, even though she
knows—she tests my eyes—that she is not going to get well.
It is such a relief, she says, not having to pretend any more.
It was so hard, more than she could bear for a very long time,
being alone with the knowledge of it.

"Had you no one to turn to?"

"No one. After I was ill I had to stay with my parents
again, you see, and my father wouldn't hear of it."

"But, your mother?"

"He insisted on protecting her, you see."

"So you knew that he knew, and still—?"

"No one would let me talk about it. It was a horrible
secret that everyone knew and no one would mention. And
the worst of it was being so helpless, a burden on everyone.
It was like having to be a child again, only worse, because
they would say, soon you will be getting stronger—and this
time, I could not. So I let them down, again and again, and
I could see them actually hating me for it despite themselves.
Then I started hating myself. Until I came here, I used to
hope each night that I wouldn't wake up to live another day.
Each hour seemed like a week, each day was like months.
And when I was in the other hospital, I had to have morphine
shots to knock me out for the pain, but that isn't living. When
it is that way, you really can't call it being alive. The psychiatrist at the other hospital was very kind and he tried to help
me, but he couldn't give me what I needed."

"Then it is very different here, for you?"

"Here I am treated as a person. I have a sense of my—
dignity. Well, I don't mean that, it sounds so proud, but here
I am simply myself, and no one minds. I am glad to live each
day now, one at a time. I like to nap in the afternoons, but I
am so busy here, it is actually hard for me to fit that in. So

many people—friends I didn't know cared for me, people I used to work with—have written to me, come to visit me and so forth, now that I am here and it is all right to say what is happening."

"How long have you been here?"

"Nine, ten weeks I think. Perhaps longer, I don't remember. It's strange, I hardly even remember the pain. I remember the fact that it was so bad, I could not bear it. . . . Yes, it was physical pain, and also the sense of being such a failure, having lost out on everything I tried to do. And the grief of losing the one child, the only thing that mattered. The pain was terrible, but I think it was grief that always made it past bearing. I was angry too. At the world and at life, and most of all, at myself. And then I came here—have you seen how it is when we come? When we arrive? Matron comes straight into the ambulance, the moment it stops in front of the door. She does that for everyone. And she came in to me, and called me by name. I looked at her face and could see that she was glad to have me. It seemed as if she had been waiting, only for me. That is why I am always so near to tears here, it is such a relief. And all that time, I never believed in God. Can you imagine? Listen, a week ago something happened that was very strange. I felt in the night the Angel of Death, it seemed. In my sleep. It was the presence of death just by my shoulder and I thought, this is my time to go. But it was not. It was the woman in the bed just there beside me, she, who died that night. But I felt it, and I went up out of my body and floated above it. I knew I was in my spiritual body then, and I was not afraid, but I was glad to come back because I am still not ready. I have to work through things in my own mind that are not finished yet. Here at the hospice, you see, things are so different from all that I am used to. I have to go over my whole life again, it seems, sorting it out. Do you think that is strange?

"You don't," she continues. "Well, that is one reason why it is so good to be here, where no one thinks I have gone mad. Let me show you something—I hope you don't mind this—but I want to show you what it was like before." She pulls back the sleeves of her nightgown and holds her arms up to the light. The scars I have seen, but never like this. Most people, when they cut their wrists, only want to bleed a little and frighten the people around them into being kinder. Lillian Preston has savaged herself, wanting to die.

"I did that," she says, shaking her head in wonder, putting her arms back under the coverlet again. "It never did heal right."

"When was it?"

"Before I came here. They sent me to one hospital, then to another. Then, when I finally came to St. Christopher's, the young man—you know, the chaplain's assistant—he came to me and we talked about it all. He helped me."

She closes her eyes and lies very still, smiling slightly, pregnant with her own death, pondering her memories, biding her time.

II
A Child Dies
ANONYMOUS

So I'll tell you my experience, it's very personal, it's a mother's feelings and it was kind of stupid, of how filled with hope we were. Our daughter was diagnosed eighteen months before she died as having myocardiopathy. Our doctor was a man of great hope, and of course you don't have to give a parent much hope. They just take the first straw of hope that's there and they just run off with it and with me I could really build a straw of hope into an oak tree. I was very optimistic. You just never think it's going to happen to you. In fact you don't even think of a child dying. She was in the hospital and on the second night I was at home with my husband and I remember saying, "You don't think she could die do you?" He answered me with, "You don't think she could do you?" and really that was the first time we had approached it and really that wasn't much of an approach because we both just dropped it. I really don't think that my husband and I lack in communication, that just goes to show that we really were filled with hope. Well, when our daughter did die she was never termed a terminal patient. She didn't have leukemia, she didn't have a brain tumor. Really no medical person could say "Your daugh-

---

The mother of the child who died gave this story to Joseph Fischhoff, M.D., Professor of Child Psychiatry at Wayne State University in Detroit, Michigan, and Noreen Brohl, M.S.W., formerly Instructor in Social Work, Department of Pediatrics, Wayne State University.

Excerpted with permission from *Journal of Pediatrics 88:* 140-146, 1976; copyrighted by The C. V. Mosby Company, St. Louis, Missouri, U.S.A.

ter is terminal" because she could go on. And of course I just
took that aspect of it. I stayed the first night with her. I was
there about twenty-four hours. I came back that Friday morning. There were some delays early in the morning so I guess
I wasn't there as early as I wanted. It was really late. She was
always very considerate of me. She never really reproached
me. She never really reproached anyone even when she was
in pain. And she had a lot of suffering for that last month. So
that morning I came in with my usual rah rah attitude, you
know, "what can I do to make you happy today" and entertain
the mind. She was a child, and I was aware that I had to keep
her mind busy. She did very well in school. In April or May,
she had taken an IQ test, the computer just ran out of paper
it was so high. But she was just a regular kid, so I was always
thinking of things to keep her up, because I knew she was
down. I turned on the TV and she said, "Mom, I want you to
hold me," and I did. She was in my arms and she wasn't
interested in the TV so we turned it off. Then she said, "I
have to get back in bed to find a place to breathe better." She
had been in an oxygen tent and it frustrated her so much. I
think that day she was allowed a few minutes out of it and I
started reading aloud, and I said let's read *Winnie the Pooh*,
one of her favorite books. I started out and she said she wanted
me to hold her again. Of course what we were going through
were her stages of congestive heart failure. I had heard that
the child starts going into a fetal position to make himself
more comfortable to breathe. She started calling for more oxygen. Then I realized she was going through the oppression
that one might feel when they are going to die, and of course
she wanted the only thing in the world that counted, her mother
to hold her and be close to her. But I wasn't picking this up
and I just wasn't picking up the signals until I saw her moving
around and calling for the oxygen. Then the nurse came and
turned up the oxygen. My daughter called for more and the
nurse came back and said, "It doesn't go up any further," and
she heard this and she looked up at me and said, "I'm going
to die. Am I going to die?" She asked me the question and
answered it herself so really she kind of prepared me. And of
course I figured out times afterward what I wasn't aware of.

So then I started talking to her. I made up a story of long lost words and perhaps since she had asked the question and she had answered it, I figured that was it, and we were both in the same boat of knowledge. I told her she was God's child, that He had just given her to us as a loan to take care of as best we could, that He wanted her back and that He was really the one who made her and loved her and He was going to take care of her, and I talked to her about this for quite a while. This is a child, remember, who was not in a coma, who died with the brain going right to the last minute, and absorbed everything, and when the audio was going I knew she could still hear me so I had until 1:25 to say something that would go with her into eternity. I really felt that she prayed. She listened to everything I said. She said three sentences that have comforted me and will comfort me until the day I die and I hope I will say the same three sentences when I die. This was a beautiful thing for a mother. She said, "I love you God, I'm sorry for my sins, and please don't let me die." I didn't realize she had any concept of sin but this is all part of training, but the fact she said I love you, God, first, and she was really short of breath. I held her for about an hour and I held her a long time after she died and nobody made me budge. I stayed in that room with her about forty or fifty minutes after she died and it was really neat. But my little girl did have a message. She has a message for me, she has a message for everybody here: the only thing when the chips are down that really matters is kindness. That's the only thing that matters. You can spell it anyway you want. Some people say love, some say compassion but when you act it out what is it, it's kindness, and that's the only thing you can give to this person that's dying. She didn't need anymore needles, anymore tests, or anymore anything. What she did ask, was for me just to be with her and hold her, and that's the message. When the chips are down what else have you got—it's one human being communicating with another and it's time to get that person ready for the absolute. It depends on your faith, I guess. I'm not sure. That's all I have to say, just be kind. And to you who are professionals, to you who have been in this hospital all day long with sick kids and dying kids, I know you have to go home at night and live with yourself and your own family and it's hard. I know you have to turn it off but please, in educating yourself to turn it off, so you can carry on your normal life and carry on functions that you have to do, please don't stifle your compassions, or your kindness.

III
Ten Bad Days Among the Dying
B. D. COLEN

One Sunday evening last May, a thirty-one-year-old man com-
plaining of violent stomach pain and vomiting was brought
by his cousin to the emergency room of the Royal Victoria
Hospital in Montreal. The hospital's chief of surgery had called
the emergency room shortly before the man's arrival and had
reported the man was on his way, might be suffering from an
intestinal blockage and was said to be dying of cancer of the
pancreas.

The physicians on duty that night had no reason to doubt
the surgeon's assessment: Their new patient was about twenty
pounds underweight; he had scars indicating he had undergone several biopsies; his skin had telltale signs of radiation
treatment. In addition, he was cold and clammy, in need of a
bath and had a patchy, four-day growth of stubble.

The young man said he was a high school teacher from
Connecticut paying what he knew would be a final visit to his
Canadian cousin when he became violently ill. He gave the
admitting physician a stack of medical records from Yale New
Haven Hospital, all of which attested to his disease and the
hopelessness of his condition, and a set of X-rays of his can-
cerous pancreas. The young man explained he had the records

Mr. Colen is author of the book Karen Ann Quinlan: Dying
in the Age of Eternal Life, *and a member of the metropolitan
staff of* The Washington Post.

Printed in *The Washington Post* Outlook section, October 14, 1976. Reprinted with permission.

with him in case he did become ill, and no one questioned the explanation.

The man told the attending physician that he had already undergone chemotherapy—with horrendous side effects and no success—and did not want any further treatment for his cancer. All he wanted, he said, was relief from the stomach pain. As preparations were made to move the new patient to a holding ward, he underwent a series of standard tests, including a blood workup.

When physicians checked the results of the blood tests they found an indication that the young man might be suffering from pancreatitis, an inflammation of the pancreas not uncommon among patients with cancer of the pancreas. They were neither surprised nor alarmed by the finding, for it only confirmed what the young man, and his medical records, had told them. So they gave the patient a shot of Demerol for his pain and had him moved to a holding ward for the night.

But as Robert W. Buckingham III, which was the patient's real name and not the one he gave upon admission, lay in the darkened Montreal hospital ward, he had to struggle to fight off a growing sense of dread and panic. For he did not expect the blood tests, or any other tests, to turn up indication of disease. As far as Buckingham knew, he was in perfect health, although incredibly tense and nervous.

Buckingham is, as he told the physicians, a teacher. But he is a doctoral teaching fellow at Yale and not a high school teacher. As a medical anthropologist, his primary job is that of evaluation coordinator for the New Haven Hospice, an institution dedicated to the care and comfort of the terminally ill. Like the staff members of hospices in Great Britain, the physicians, nurses, social workers and volunteers at the New Haven Hospice are carers, rather than curers. Their principal goal is to free terminal patients of debilitating pain to enable them to live out the days prior to their deaths.

And there he was, only a few hours into what was revealed Wednesday as one of the most successful, painstakingly constructed deceptions in the annals of anthropological research, and already it seemed as though something might be going wrong. It turned out that Buckingham was simply suffering a stress reaction, but he says he could never repeat the ten gut-wrenching days he spent "living with the dying," observing and chronicling the actions and interactions, social relations and hierarchical structures among staff members, terminal patients and relatives of the terminally ill, studying them in much the same way anthropologists have long studied the cultures of various native peoples.

Because of what he saw as the practical impossibility of gathering data about the lives of the dying and their caretakers by observing them, Buckingham arranged to live among the patients as a patient. He was aided in his deception by the physicians, who provided him with a bogus medical history, and by his colleagues at the New Haven Hospice. The director of the Royal Victoria, the hospital attorney, the chief of surgery and the medical director of the hospice unit in the hospital were all aware of Buckingham's mission. None of the patients or staff members in the units was told anything about the study.

During his two days in the holding unit, four days on a surgical care ward and four days on a hospice or palliative care ward, Buckingham was able to document much of the insensitivity medical science has long accorded those who are beyond its help. And he was able to prove his assumptions about the efficacy of the hospice system of care for the hopelessly ill.

Buckingham took copious notes during the ten days in the hospital, telling anyone who asked that he was writing a book and "wanted to finish before I died." The only person who commented about his note taking, he said, was a nurse who said, "I hope you're not writing about this hospital."

The results of Buckingham's research, contained in a paper to be published by the Canadian Medical Association Journal, are interesting, though hardly startling.

He found, for instance, that while he was visited virtually the same number of times by staff members on the surgical ward and staff members on the hospice ward, the mean number of minutes per contact was 5.5 on the surgical unit and nineteen in the hospice. Nurses in the surgical unit spent 2.4

mean minutes per contact with Buckingham, while the hospice nurses spent a mean of thirteen minutes per contact.

"Patients, in general, experienced monotony and loneliness on the surgical ward," he wrote in his paper, while "kindness and individual attention were a matter of policy and the system facilitated these attributes" in the hospice unit.

"[I] heard laughter for the first time two days after . . . admission. A student nurse was talking to an elderly man. She took a personal interest in the patients and spoke with openness about herself and the hospital. The only staff groups who initiated conversations were the student nurses and orderlies. Personal requests made to other staff were frequently ignored or forgotten."

The surgical ward, Buckingham concluded, is solely designed for the care of the body, while the needs of the spirit are ignored. Buckingham's "overall impression was that the surgical ward had highly developed skills in acute care. The staff displayed great efficiency in preparing patients for surgery and caring for them post-operatively."

In the hospice, or palliative care unit (PCU), Buckingham found the same kind of highly developed technical skills, but he writes that they were balanced by a humane touch missing on the surgery unit.

"On arrival at the palliative care ward [I] found some flowers and a card by [my] bedside saying, 'Welcome, Mr. M.' (Buckingham refers to himself as Mr. M. throughout the paper.) The initial nursing interview was conducted by a nurse who introduced herself by name, sat down so that her eyes were on a level with [mine] and proceeded to listen. There was no hurry, her questions flowed from [my] previous answers, and there was acceptance of the expressions of [my] own concerns. She asked such questions as, 'What do you like to eat?' and, 'Is there anything special you like to do?'

"In [my] first few hours on the palliative care ward, [I] observed that the professionalism of the staff members was balanced by a notable freedom to express their own personality. This contrasted with the behavior on the surgical care ward where the smiles were rare and personalities hidden . . . On the surgical care ward direct orders to patients were commonplace, whereas they never occurred on the palliative care ward. All these details conveyed a 'happy spirit' and 'an attitude of caring' that was sensed and commented on by the patients."

FAMILY ROLES

One of the aspects of life in both wards which Buckingham observed most carefully was the role of patients' families in patient care.

"Relatives suffered from physicians' inaccessibility on the surgical ward," he wrote. "Queries on medications, diet and many other topics were always referred to the doctor, and in his absence they were left unanswered . . . When the patient is clearly improving, such ignorance may be bearable. When a loved one is daily deteriorating, much better communication is necessary. In addition, families need an outlet for grief, help with their own fear, loss, resentments, anger, guilt and other common emotions. They need to begin to plan to fill the role of the dying person in the family.

"On the palliative care ward [I] observed relatives inquiring for the doctor five times. On each occasion the doctor was reached and either came or spoke to the family on the phone. In addition, nurses, volunteers and other staff members were willing and allowed to answer queries.

"The visitors' room was a vital space on surgery," wrote Buckingham, "where families felt at ease and gathered to give each other support. They sensed they were in the way at the bedside. On the PCU, the TV lounge was important, but families also spent much time at the bedside participating in the care of the patient. They changed bed linen, washed and fed the patient, brought the urinal, plumped the pillows frequently. The staff encouraged the family to experience the meaning of death by allowing them to help in the care of the dying."

ETHICAL QUESTIONS

Robert Buckingham's sojourn among the dying began with a

lighthearted remark. As he remembers it now, one day in May, 1975, Buckingham, Dr. Sylvia Lack, medical director of the New Haven Hospice, and Dr. Balfour Mont, medical director of the Royal Victoria Hospice, were discussing the difficulty of gathering data to confirm their belief that a hospice setting afforded the dying patient superior care.

"What you're really trying to do is evaluate the quality of care, aren't you?" Buckingham remembers asking the two doctors. "Bal Mont said, 'Yes,' and I kiddingly suggested they bring in a pseudo patient."

To prepare for his hospital stay Buckingham "just stopped eating" and dropped twenty pounds from his already spare frame. He underwent ultraviolet exposure to simulate radiation treatment, and he had a cooperative surgeon perform the minor operation needed to produce the "biopsy" scars. There were also various "stress reactions" Buckingham hadn't planned on.

"I got plantar warts, psoriasis and five weeks of impotence." When asked last week if all the side effects had cleared up, he said, laughing, "No, but the impotence has cleared up and that's the only one I really cared about."

While Buckingham can laugh a little about some of his experiences, he says he is more nervous now, as he awaits the medical and anthropological community's reaction to his study and the deception he employed, than he was about going into the hospital. And he has good reason to be nervous.

Once widely accepted, the ethics of so-called clandestine participant observation—which some would call spying—are being called into question more and more in almost direct relationship to the stress being put upon the need always to obtain consent from patients, or other participants, in such research.

"The underlying ethical question," said Dr. Robert M. Veatch when told of Buckingham's project, "is whether the fact that you can't get the data any other way justifies the deception. The feeling more and more," said Veatch, a fellow at the Institute of Society, Ethics and the Life Sciences at Hastings-on-Hudson, N.Y., "is that it's not." Veatch went on to say that he has no doubt that a study such as Buckingham's,

as it was explained to Veatch, would not meet the guidelines
for informed consent required for any project using Department of Health, Education and Welfare monies. While they
did not discuss the HEW guidelines, Dr. Lack and Buckingham were very careful to stress that Buckingham, who is
paid for his regular work with federal funds, was on leave
without pay while preparing the study.

LIVING THE ROLE

Whether or not Buckingham's work is enthusiastically received in the academic community, it represents an effort he
says he could never repeat.

"It's not worth doing again. It's not worth the wear and
tear on me and on my relations with people and my anxiety.
The findings were worth doing it once. It would destroy
[someone who tried to do it repeatedly]. I could have held on
maybe five days more; I could have struggled through it. But
I was so glad to get out of there, even to get out of the great
PCU."

Buckingham said that while he was in the PCU he began
to experience "excruciating pain, real pain and I was weak.
I couldn't eat." He had so psyched himself into the role of the
terminal patient that he began to live the role. Dr. Elisabeth
Kübler-Ross, author of the renowned book, *On Death and
Dying,* and a believer in the theory that some cancers are psychosomatically induced, is worried for Buckingham.

"She said that because I put myself in a role, and accepted that role, I went through what we call in the field
identity transferral—I really believed I was sick. I took the
role of a patient. I was lonely, I was depressed." Kübler-Ross
fears that Buckingham could have stepped permanently over
the threshold from one role into another.

"She feels your mind controls your body, and I come
from a cancer-prone family. She is very concerned. It's the
only thing she is concerned about [in regard to] the study. I'm
in the field I am because my mother died of cancer six years
ago. We do things for personal and professional reasons."

ASSESSMENT OF DEATH

Having lived among the dying, would it be easier for Buckingham to have to face an early death, or more difficult?

"It's going to be easier. Working with these people, and seeing the sense of love and meshing together of people and people rallying around one another, not because of social status, just because they're people—it's a beautiful thing. I thought about this: If I did die now would I be angry about it? And the answer would be no. I'd be better prepared because I saw what people go through. I'm not predicting my reaction, but . . .

"I think I could handle it. In many ways I'm more prepared. I have the role behavior already," said Buckingham.

"How has this made you rethink your own mortality?" he was asked.

"Well, I thought dying young would be a shame. But if you work with the dying, you look at your life a bit differently. Things that seemed important before are not as important as they were. There's a whole sense of softness, almost. The way you look at trees and flowers and people as people.

"If one lives life to one's fullest, if one can go to bed at night and say, 'Was today a good day, would I be prepared to die tomorrow?' and the answer is yes, I would be prepared to die. I would not be afraid to die. I would want as little indignity as possible. This has brought me closer to death. It has made me stronger, and made me better able to cope with my own life. You learn a lot about life through the dying."

But as much as he says he has learned and grown through his work, Buckingham stresses the fact that what he did was a one-time-only experiment. "You know," he said with an ironic laugh, "you can't make a living out of being terminally ill."

IV

The Doctor and the Cancer Patient
ERNEST H. ROSENBAUM, M.D.

Good health is the greatest asset we have in life. When it is impaired because of an accident or an illness such as cancer, or kidney or heart disease, we are forced to make compromises. A twenty-six-year-old woman with advanced melanoma who has made these compromises recently wrote me,

> I now see things in a much different light. Even though I probably will die young, I don't just sit around and wait for it. Actually, no one is given any more time than I am. We wake each morning to a new day, and that is all. No one is promised ahead of time that they will be here for the spring vacation, for the wedding in August, or even for the dentist appointment next Thursday. We are all equal in that we have one day to fill with anything we please. The quality of life lived each day is more important than how long we live. . . . I am not the only one in the boat but no one else can do my living or dying for me.

This woman is typical of a person who has a strong will

Dr. Rosenbaum is Associate Clinical Professor at the University of California in San Francisco, Medical Director of the San Francisco Regional Tumor Foundation, and Associate Chief of Medicine at Mount Zion Hospital and Medical Center.

This article appeared entitled "Oncology/Hematology and Psychosocial Support of the Cancer Patient," Chapter 19 by Ernest Rosenbaum in the book *Psychosocial Care of the Dying Patient,* by Charles A. Garfield.

to live, who continues to live even as she is dying. My goal as a doctor is to try to help each of my patients achieve a similar equilibrium. Sometimes I succeed, sometimes I fail; but the way I handle each patient is based on a recognition of his or her special emotional needs as well as of the terror and anxiety that are common to anyone who has been diagnosed as having a potentially fatal disease.

When a patient is referred to me for a preliminary diagnosis or for reevaluation, it does not matter whether cancer is only suspected or whether it has been a reality for some time. The anxiety of each patient is extreme, the silent questions overwhelming. To begin to penetrate this terror, I explain at our first meeting my belief that the most beneficial relationship between us must be based on mutual trust and candor. To help him face his fears and anxieties, I explain the diagnostic procedures he will undergo. I discuss the reasons for doing each test, the range of possible results, positive and negative, and I assure him that if the results are positive, we have an arsenal of therapies with which to attack his problem. Finally, I continually ask each patient whether he has any questions and urge him to write them down as they occur to him so that he will not suppress these thoughts and add to his anxiety.

When testing is completed and the results indicate a malignancy, I arrange for the patient to come to my office at a time when I will be able to explain the situation to him or her without interruption. When possible, I prefer to have the closest family members present during the explanation. This eliminates the need for repetition and reduces the possibility of a misunderstanding. The presence of a close family member or friend also helps lessen a patient's fear of abandonment and reassures him that details about his condition are not being concealed from him.

Knowing that what I say in this interview is crucial and may affect the rest of a patient's life, I proceed slowly and carefully, ready to temper my approach as he reveals how much he wants to know at that moment. Although I encourage candor and full partnership between myself and each patient, it is still a patient's prerogative to choose how much he wants to hear at any given time. I give detailed explanations of his disease, repeating much of the basic information I gave him during the diagnostic procedures. Most important, I describe the treatments that are available to combat his disease and reassure him that although we will begin with one mode of therapy, there are others that may be equally good or will provide a backup if the first one is not effective.

For the past two years, for the benefit of both patient and family, I have tape recorded these thirty-to-forty-minute initial meetings of my explanation and of their questions and reactions and given them the recording to take home. I use this form of reinforcement for two reasons. The person who has just learned he or she has a serious disease is stunned and may hear little of what I say. He is busy thinking, "Why me?" or "How much will I suffer?" or "What will happen to my family?" The cassette recording, listened to at home in a more rational moment, will provide the same vital information and give reassurance to him and his family that there are concrete medical steps that can be taken to help him. Reviewing the information in this way also helps create openness between the patient and his family about the disease and the problems they will face as well as providing a springboard for future discussions between us. Many patients have told me that this procedure has added a new dimension to their understanding of their disease and their planned program of treatment.

Occasionally a situation will arise in which a patient or a member of his family will request that I keep information from the other one. In such cases I try to convince them of the desirability of openness with each other, but if I am ever forced to take a stand, I will side with the patient (except in an extreme case where a patient suffers from severe mental or emotional problems), for it is with him that I have made my covenant for honesty. It is his battle for life with which I am concerned, his feelings, his well-being. He, not his family, has come to me for service.

One of the obvious advantages of a well-informed patient who understands all of his options is his willingness to undergo therapy. Moreover, it is absurd to think of giving complicated treatments, with their possible side effects, to someone who is uninformed.

At no time during the course of treatment, even in the earliest stages of disease and medical therapy, should the subject of pain, suffering, or death be avoided. A patient always knows whether he can broach these terrifying subjects with his doctor. He will know intuitively whether his doctor is afraid and defensive. As one of my patients said,

> It is in the earliest meetings, even before the diagnosis, that the tone of the relationship is set. In these encounters, the physician reveals his attitudes toward the disease and the patient. He establishes the foundation of confidence and support on which the patient will later rely. If he shows respect for the patient and his own courage in the face of cancer, he will immediately begin to win the patient's trust. It is important to achieve this before the diagnosis because the physician's manner in presenting the diagnosis and the patient's reaction to it have an enormous effect on the course of the disease.
>
> Having had cancer for more than two years, I know what a doctor can mean in liberating one to live actively during the remaining time of one's life. Thus, a doctor should recognize that by his own courage and respect for the patient, he can relieve terror. If he shows confidence that he can remain in control of the disease and the pain, it removes an enormous burden from the patient's life.

When the doctor is afraid, the patient is afraid and communicates this fear to his family and friends, the very people who should be enlisted to support him in his ordeal.

The successful long-term treatment of any patient will depend to a great degree on a patient's attitude. If he can strive for and maintain a positive attitude, which means he is willing to fight for his life and believes he can live longer by doing so, he very often will respond better to treatment. I remember several instances where two patients who were similar in age, diagnosis, and degree of illness, and who were undergoing the same type of treatment, had different therapeutic results. The only discernible difference between them was the pessimism of those who did less well and the optimism and determination of the others to live as fully as possible despite their debilities.

I do not believe that I can *create* a positive attitude where none has existed before, but to the extent that I must know each patient intimately in order to prescribe and regulate therapy and to give him or her emotional support, I can also encourage a positive attitude in many ways. One way is to alleviate his or her fears concerning chemotherapy. Many people have heard frightening stories from uninformed relatives and friends about the side effects of treatment, both conventional and experimental. These stories make them more afraid of therapy than they are of cancer. I assure these patients that if side effects occur, I will try to alter the therapy or the method or the time of application, not only to reduce the side effects but also to enable them to coordinate treatment with their other commitments. For example, working people can often be put on a program that does not interfere with their work schedules by receiving therapy just before the weekend. The side effects will have worn off by Monday.

Another source of anxiety and depression for a patient is his feeling of a loss of autonomy, of a new dependence on others—the medical team. From the day he seeks help for his symptoms, a person is questioned, poked, prodded, tested, and given treatment. I try to mitigate these unwelcome feelings of dependence by prescribing, when feasible, a program that includes oral chemotherapy that can be taken at home, and, in the later stages of disease, by encouraging home care and self-administered pain shots.

Fear of the unknown—of changes in therapy or of periodic test results—is always a source of acute anxiety for a cancer patient. For this reason I always describe the risks, side effects, and anticipated results of all the therapies appropriate to each person's disease in order to prevent unnecessary shocks in the present or the future. I also explain that it is not uncommon to change from one mode of therapy to another, to alter the dosage or content of a therapy, or even to cease therapy altogether for a time. I tell patients that such moves should not be misconstrued as a failure of therapy or a progression of disease. For those who worry whether their current therapy is effective, I can also reassure them that we will try something else if that one fails.

These are the kinds of anxieties that can be alleviated during regular office visits. Therefore, I encourage patients to always keep a list of questions that occur to them between visits. Many people are so fearful of receiving bad news during an office visit that they forget the worries that plagued them during the previous week or two.

Since any anxiety or worry can break down a patient's determination to fight, I also try to discern when there may be nonmedical problems that contribute to a patient's depression. The fear of losing a job, or a misunderstanding with a relative or a friend, should not be added to the ordeal of coping with cancer. I obviously cannot solve these dilemmas for my patients but I can, by listening to them, give emotional support.

Since it is not always possible to tell solely from talks during office visits what extra burdens a patient must endure in addition to cancer, I try, if requested, to make a house call early in a relationship. A very well-dressed patient may actually live in minimal circumstances or suffer from tension caused by another family member. One of my patients, a middle-aged man with colon cancer, became desperately ill one evening and finally telephoned me. I found him in a rooming house in a deteriorating part of town. He lived in one small room and shared a bathroom at the end of the hall with several other people, making colostomy care difficult when he had diarrhea. When he suffered side effects from chemotherapy, he had to depend on the manager of the rooming house to bring him his meals. He had been too proud to ask for help, but having discovered his true situation, I was able to mobilize nursing care and other assistance.

The causes of fear and anxiety and other types of problems I have mentioned all prevent a cancer patient from maintaining an attitude that will allow him to function maximally for his type and stage of disease. When these emotional problems are brought out in the open and possible remedies are discussed by doctor and patient, the patient gains a little more freedom to spend on the ordinary things of life—work, recreation, the pursuit of knowledge, the enjoyment of family and friends. It is this actuality of being able to participate in and enjoy the things one has always enjoyed that is the definition of having a positive attitude. One of my patients, a psychiatrist, is an excellent example of a person who has achieved this. He says,

> This is a very, very rich period in every single dimension of my life, whether that's family, sports, music, or my work. At least at this time I have no physical limitations and can maintain my former level of life. Cancer has not robbed or significantly diluted the capacity I have always had to enjoy life. I think most people are not transformed psychologically by having cancer, even though they may live their lives somewhat differently. Their victory is in the full continuation of their lives without being paralyzed by regressive fears and needs. Their victory is that of actively living while enduring cancer. This is made possible, in part, when doctor and patient are honest and open with each other. Then, although fears and fantasies don't disappear, they are put into a manageable perspective, and the individual is freed to do more than engage in solitary battle with his own phantoms.

Another person who approaches the problems of living with cancer in a positive manner is this woman of thirty-five, who is married and the mother of a seven-year-old girl:

> Cancer is devastating. At first you can't even think about it. You're smacked hard and all the wind goes out of you. You don't begin to think until you reach a plateau where you know you're doing well. Then you begin to think about yourself and your family and your reasons for living.
>   I've seen people destroy themselves with their attitude in all kinds of situations, and although I don't believe your attitude can cure your disease, I do believe it can help you. Therefore, I reject my negative thought. It sounds insane, but it keeps me healthy. Negative thinking breaks down my energy level. Although my drive and my will and my pace are basically the same as they were before, I have changed in one way. I no longer fly off the handle over unimportant matters. My priorities

are being alive and loving my family. I've always loved life, and the biggest pain is that I didn't have enough of it when this thing happened. So I said, "Screw you, world. I just ain't leaving."

The positive attitudes of these two patients represent what I call the *will to live,* and give a fifth dimension to the four traditional therapies—surgery, radiotherapy, chemotherapy, and experimental immunotherapy. I have said that patients with positive attitudes tend to respond better to therapy and are better able to cope with their disease-related problems. Some doctors and psychologists go further than this. They believe that the proper attitude may even have an effect upon cell function and consequently may be utilized to arrest, if not cure, cancer. In an effort to support their views, they are conducting studies to determine to what extent the mind and emotions are involved either as a contributing factor in the onset of cancer or as a means of altering its course.

Some researchers are exploring the possibility that people with certain personality traits may be more susceptible to developing cancer. Others are experimenting with methods of actively enlisting the mind in the body's combat with cancer, and to this end techniques such as meditation, biofeedback, and visualization are being employed. (Visualization involves the creation in a patient's mind of positive images about what is occurring in the body.) At present doctors and patients are divided on this issue of the degree of influence of mind over body. Personally, I do not think that any of the studies that have so far been conducted are scientifically valid. There is as yet no proof that a person can control his cancer with his mind. One of my patients, cured of leukemia, vigorously disagrees, however, and will not to this day even acknowledge that chemotherapy was the agent that pulled him through. He says,

Chemotherapy was a crutch and I was willing to go along with all the crutches. I was willing to use any means available until I was able to do it myself. I don't respect it [cancer] at all because the moment I do, I'll be afraid of it, and fear is the greatest enemy in this thing. . . .

Every disease, though real, is psychosomatically induced. There are no exceptions. The emotional and mental state of the individual triggers the germs and viruses in the body that cause disease. . . . I also subscribe to the notion that anything can be done if you believe in it strongly enough, and that includes the eradication of disease.

A second patient believes, as I do, that although a person cannot use his mind to effect a cure, a good attitude is still very important.

Having acute leukemia in 1975 is somewhat akin to having the Black Plague in 1340 in Europe—namely, that one has no idea what the causality of it is. This can encourage magical thinking that somehow one has done something to provoke the forces of nature and that one only need do something else to regain control over them. This is the most fearsome thing to me—one's complete helplessness before the forces of nature. It would naturally be comforting to believe you brought about your cancer by your own emotions, actions, or state of mind. Scientifically, there may be some basis for believing that the emotional state has something to do with a person's response to cancer, but if the emotions do play a role, I don't think it's an obvious or a major one. On the other hand, I am certain that trying to maintain a state of psychological well-being won't hurt.

When I speak of the will to live, I don't mean some kind of simple, blind faith or optimism. To me it has more to do with the kind of stance or posture that one adopts toward the disease, namely an aggressive, fighting posture. Having an attitude of doing battle with the disease and having some knowledge of the drugs, the program, and so on, makes it easier to cope with the discomfort because one then understands what is going on.

It will be many years before we know whether it is possible for the mind to control the immune defense system. In the meantime, the experiments of biofeedback and visualization are helpful to patients in that they encourage positive thinking and provide relaxation. However, these methods can also be damaging when a patient puts all his or her faith in them or ignores conventional therapy. For instance, in one of the current philosophies, Carl Simonton, M.D.,[1] tells patients that they have unconsciously brought on their disease and that they have the power within them to decide whether they will live or die by changing their beliefs and improving their self-image. Through visualization the patient is taught to relax and mentally picture his disease, with the white blood cells attacking and overcoming the cancer cells. While such a procedure can lift a depressed patient who needs hope or a way to help himself, it can also prove psychologically devastating if he totally accepts the thesis that he has brought on all his discomfort and pain through his own personality and stressful way of life. The extreme guilt, disappointment—and often bitterness—when the disease progresses would not be necessary if realistic, rather than false, hope were given before participation in the program. Visualization is still in the theoretical stages. Perhaps it will turn out to be true that we cause our own cancer, but to create guilt and remorse before proof exists is a mistake, however well-intentioned and devoted the advocates of the theory.

My criticism is limited, however, for I do appreciate that these methods can increase the will to live and I recommend them to my patients. I also suggest to patients that they can, if they feel the need, avail themselves of one of the psychiatric support programs of private counseling or group therapy that are offered by a variety of institutions: hospitals; major cancer treatment centers; social welfare departments; and the American Cancer Society. Sharing frustrations with others in similar circumstances often relieves the sense of isolation that cancer patients experience. I think that none of us, even if we have been dangerously ill, can have any concept of the depths of despair and terror that are experienced by a person who has a terminal disease.

Thus, it is understandable why people grasp at straws.

As cancer advances, the emotional and mental assaults increase, seriously compromising a person's self-image. After all, a sense of worth is directly related to what we do and how we interact with others. For instance, when a cancer patient is unable to work as hard as he did before his illness, or has less energy for family activities than he used to, he has feelings of shame and guilt. If his disease is terminal, his sense of being defective and even somehow to blame for his condition may be intensified. Unfortunately, these feelings of impotence and isolation are corroborated and reinforced by others in the worst way, for cancer does, unfortunately, make many people uncomfortable. Some even think it is infectious. The cancer patient of today has been equated with the leper of yesterday, so often does he encounter fear and avoidance in family and friends, nurses and doctors.

These attitudes contribute to psychological deterioration, which is intensified by the patient's awareness of his bodily deterioration. The paradox is that the more physically dependent on others he becomes, the more psychologically and emotionally cut off he is. To better understand these devastating aspects of living with cancer, I sometimes tape record conversations with selected individuals who want to contribute their thoughts and feelings to help others. One such person is Dr. Arnon Fortgang,[2] a surgeon in San Francisco who describes what happened following his own diagnosis of cancer.

Cancer, while a dreaded illness, does not necessarily totally immobilize the patient, nor render him an invalid. A decrease in productivity, however, can occur for various reasons. There is some physical weakness and increased fatigue, as well as some reduced drive and initiative. In addition, there are fewer opportunities open to the cancer patient—and very often he is not given an opportunity to return to his previous job or profession. Our society, which professes the need for rehabilitation and reconstitution of the injured or ill, tends, in reality, to shut the cancer patient out of the mainstream of his usual employment, severely curbing his productivity. This takes the form of inaccessibility to the previous job.

In the case of professionals, such as self-employed physicians, medical practice becomes impractical because of current exorbitant malpractice insurance fees, hospital rules, and disability schedules that do not allow for partial disability ratings. Thus, the medical cancer patient is often prevented from returning to work and similar experiences are common among cancer patients in other professions.

There are also changes in the relationship between the cancer patient and his peers. Either there is a taboo around him, or his more enlightened friends may show empathy and sympathy, which usually stem from the attitude that "if it happened to him it could happen to me." Nevertheless, while there is a considerable amount of personal empathy and sympathy, there is as yet no organized structure geared to the rehabilitation and return to normalcy for the cancer patient. This situation creates, for the patient, a feeling of partial death. He is not wanted on the job, on committees, or on boards. His office starts looking like a morgue—full of old records and X-rays, but no new activity. What soon dawns on the patient is that he has been compromised over and over again. Initially, there is an illness that tends to render him less effective, on top of which there are limitations on his working opportunities. This often results in being offered a lesser job than he had before. Thus, while the illness itself forces him to compromise once, the other factors force him to compromise over and over again.

As a cancer patient you try your darndest, every waking minute, to stay on top of your tragedy. Then you encounter these powerful negating roadblocks that counteract all your efforts. What is so painful about all of this is that although you cannot do much about being ill, you can sustain yourself by deciding to go back to work and be productive in the field in which you are trained. And yet, there are these external barriers that deprive you of what is most important to you and that become the most disabling feature of your illness. You get a feeling of running into a solid brick wall—total frustration.

In recent years a considerable body of evidence has accumulated that the mind has the capacity to have a positive effect in illness on body healing, body resistance to tumor, and body ability to develop immunity to tumors. By not being able to do one's work and to use one's mind positively, however, a double evil emerges. Because of the illness a person is limited generally, and on top of it he is rendered ineffective by forced compromises in work. Thus the mind, which could have a beneficial effect, is not allowed to fulfil its positive function in the struggle with the illness. Enforced idleness promotes depression that in turn reduces the will to live. What can be done about all of this? Rehabilitation concepts similar to ones used in other disabilities have to be applied to the cancer patient. There are certainly no simple solutions. If the patient has a long-range, guaranteed remission, the possibilities of retraining can be considered even though this might need subsidizing from outside sources. If the remission is short or uncertain then the only acceptable solution would be that of being absorbed into the old job or profession. This might need special consideration initially in regard to financial help. There should be provisions for part-time work and allowances for partial disability to encourage the return to work. Unfortunately, a more practical solution is to accept a lesser job that requires less training than a person has had, and even a lesser income. This is a poor solution. It is a forced compromise on an already compromised patient. Such a setback would be difficult for a healthy person to accept and tolerate; it is even more difficult for a person who is ill.

As Dr. Fortgang says, there are no simple solutions. Fortunately, many patients are able to return to their jobs after the initial discovery and treatment of their disease. In the process of adjusting to living with cancer and returning to active living, they may receive help from doctors, nurses, social workers, or clergy; or from people associated with special organizations such as the American Cancer Society (including its Reach to Recovery Program), the United Ostomy Association, or the International Association of Laryngectomies.

If a person's disease becomes progressively worse, however, he or she will eventually experience all the depressing situations described by Dr. Fortgang. He will be forced to

change his work or to work fewer hours; he will find that
many people are uncomfortable in his presence. He will feel
his sense of inner dignity and self-respect have been irretriev-
ably compromised. And, in addition to these emotional strug-
gles, he will not only feel physically weak from his disease
but may also experience unpleasant side effects from radiotherapy or chemotherapy. Side effects unquestionably make
some days worse than others for some people. If we knew in
advance who was going to benefit from treatment, and who
was not, we could spare the latter group the ordeal of unpleasant side effects, but doctors are not prophets, and the per-
centages in favor of another remission indicate in most cases
that further treatment is desirable.

One patient, however, who had a particularly bad time
with chemotherapy, described it as follows:

> It's an indescribably awful experience. It's like going
> every morning and having an injection of stomach flu.
> You do it every morning, and you do it yourself. It isn't
> like, "If I'd only worn boots, I wouldn't have caught
> stomach flu." You're going out to be whipped every day.
> You think people get depressed or are cowards because
> they're not willing to take it. But, goddammit, it takes
> away from you. When I think of the things I've gone
> through, I'm appalled. I don't know where I found the
> resources. I've got to be satisfied that I can still live with
> quality. I think treatment risks doing a great disservice
> to people who want not to be bothered anymore. But that
> isn't the same as folding up with no hope and going into
> a catatonic state, waiting to die. That's obviously one
> kind of reaction. But there are a whole bunch of people
> who just don't want to futz around anymore. They want
> to do their thing and then they want to drop dead. But
> treatment does terrible things. I could talk about the in-
> jections and get sick—actually throw up thinking about
> them—even though I haven't had them lately. A cerebral
> person like me doesn't want to be tied to a bodily func-
> tion that affects his mind. The point is that you really
> change.

The results of this man's treatment were only fair, since

chemotherapy merely slowed down the growth of his tumor. But his side effects were out of proportion to the strength of the drug, a reaction I attribute to anxiety. The anticipation of bad results from a previous negative experience can actually increase toxicity. This case is a good example of why I feel I must be flexible and treat each person individually, and, at the same time, be ready to discern when a therapeutic change may have a good psychological effect. When a person is discouraged and depressed from the side effects of chemotherapy or from the routine of treatment, I sometimes suggest stopping therapy for a short time. This will at least give him a rest, and, because he feels better, it may also give him the impetus to travel, to work on an important project, or to participate more fully in family activities.

When a person is in an advanced state of decline, however, a change or cessation of therapy may provide only small respite. During this stage of an illness, the pressures on both patient and family are manifold. For this reason I urge them to continue their policy of candor with each other and with me concerning their feelings, fears, and questions. I remind them of the emotional relief that comes from frank talk, that they will be freed from the strain of hiding their own feelings while trying to guess what every other person is thinking and feeling. Fears and frustrations can then be dealt with as they arise and not left to fester until they become too overwhelming to mention, or until the habit of withholding evolves into irretrievable isolation.

The candor I advocate between a patient and his or her family and friends includes a recognition of each other's needs as well as fears. Family members have a need to give, to feel they are doing something practical to contribute to the recovery or comfort of their loved one, whether he be at home or in the hospital. The separation caused by the hospitalization of the cancer patient is particularly traumatic. The wife or husband, child or parent, leaves the hospital each evening and worries whether his or her loved one will ever again lead a normal life or even leave the hospital. Feeling impotent, these family members need to give of themselves. Fortunately, there are many practical services they can perform for the patient while he or she is in the hospital—services such as feeding, walking, turning, and massaging. I encourage this kind of active participation because these acts, along with the offer of special foods or a favorite pillow, give solace to family and patient alike.

When a patient is at home, there are also many opportunities for the members of the family to give emotional support through practical means. For example, a patient may be anxious about his next visit to the doctor, wondering whether a new problem will be discovered or a new treatment recommended. He may not have transportation to and from the doctor's office or he may dread the side effects from the day's treatment. A spouse, parent, or friend can offer him a ride or accompany him on the bus; if they are working and unable to help in this way, they can still be present to give comfort and support in the evening when the patient may have to endure the side effects of therapy.

To be realistic, however, not every family is able to be open, loving, or intelligently supportive in the manner I have described, before or after a crisis. Even those people who have always assumed their family relationships were stable may find their traditional harmony is severely threatened by the pressures of a long-term illness. Under the strain of worry and fear, latent problems may emerge among those caring for the patient. Formerly controlled anger or guilt may surface in a sudden verbal attack upon him, or in indifferent or oversolicitous behavior toward him. The exhaustion and frustration of constant worry can break the most loyal supporter. I have also seen the most courageous of patients break under these pressures. When a person has fought long and hard against cancer, lost and regained hope many times, and then realizes the battle is not to be won, he often experiences a rage and depression that seek as their target the nearest available person—spouse, child, parent, or the nurse on duty. The anger is usually manifested as irritation over a trivial matter that in normal times would not even concern the patient. When these situations arise, I try to make the person under attack—patient or family member or friend—understand that this is not a rejection of him or her but a cry of anguish.

A cancer patient must also endure the endless boredom of being ill, as well as the fear of being a burden—the latter at a time when he or she wants and needs special attention. Unfortunately, the people from whom he needs this attention are also suffering from the tedium of the day-to-day routine of illness or, as I have mentioned, from feelings of inadequacy and guilt at not being able to relieve the patient's suffering. Unable to face the reality in which the patient is imprisoned, their attention diminishes, and the patient experiences added bitterness and increasing feelings of loneliness.

Even when these dire situations do not arise, when family and friends are candid, loving, and supportive, the cancer patient is alone in much of his physical and mental suffering, in his knowledge that death is not far off. Although the devastating experience of gaining and losing hope is shared by family and friends, it is actually lived by the patient in a way none of us can know until we experience it ourselves. The same forty-five-year-old man who described his reactions to chemotherapy, also described to me, upon his return from a business trip to Alaska, this experience of uncertainty and repeated loss of hope:

I've seen any number of pictures of the tundra and the arctic wastes, but until I was up there I had not visualized how frightening; how truly frightening it is to be up there. The size is beyond conception. It isn't like the photographs, with borders. It's without borders. It's without words. I chartered a small plane and flew across the north slope for hundreds of miles. There is nothing—no life, no polar bears, just snow. You can walk for eighteen hundred miles over the pole and down into Siberia. There is just nothing out there. I thought of the foolishness—or the incredible bravery—of the men in 1903 who started out across the ice cover, risking death. I've been close to death, but it's one thing to be there all of a sudden and not to whimper, and it's another to march across a plain resolutely, knowing that when you get there, you drop off. And it's another yet to know that you are marching across the plain to the edge, but kind of blindfolded so that you get to see only occasionally.

Treatment is that experience. It's marching across a plain resolutely, sometimes blindfolded, which is when you are receiving treatment or are in a remission or whatever, but sometimes just seeing that you are getting closer. Suddenly the blindfold comes off and you are really close and it comes as a surprise. That is why people become freaked by their experience with treatment. And that's how people break. It's the uncertainty. There are lots of people who could march out there with certainty and with dignity. But there will be a breakthrough on the horizon, which is now so close, and it will suddenly be extended—perhaps to infinity. How many times can people take that? I don't think I can take it, and I consider myself a very strong person.

Thus, in the case of terminal illness, a patient suffers far more than physical deterioration. We have heard from the patients themselves what it is like to be forced into semiretirement, to lose their self-respect, to experience the discomfort of others in their presence, to gain and lose hope for recovery. As the twenty-six-year-old girl said, "I am not the only one in the boat, but no one else can do my living or dying for me." The only thing a doctor or nurse, a husband, wife, child, or friend can do, is to *be* there, to communicate freely, and to show compassion.

None of us should add to the loneliness of a dying person by refusing to acknowledge what is happening to him or her. I emphasize this because the question so often arises as to whether a doctor should tell a patient when he is dying. The results of a recent study cited by John Hunt, M.D.,[3] at a conference in England in March 1975, illustrate the inappropriateness of such a question. The study revealed that 70 percent of doctors did not want to tell the truth while 80 percent of the patients expressed a desire to know what was happening to them. My own policy at such a time is the same as it was in the days of the diagnosis. I encourage discussion and candor. I let a patient know I am willing to answer all his questions, but I also try to be sensitive to his feelings and his ability to deal with bad news on any given day. The truth must not be allowed to extinguish realistic hope, even though that hope may extend no further than the next month or next week. Candor and the will to live must coexist in a delicate balance. When that balance is tipped and a patient is deprived of hope, the results are no different than if he had been the victim of a voodoo curse. In most cases his subsequent decline is inexplicably rapid. Thus, the will to live, the fifth dimension of cancer therapy, is as important to a patient's emotional and physical well-being at this time as it is in the months and years when he is actively living with his disease.

I almost always discuss with a patient every aspect of his or her condition during this period. We talk about when to stop anticancer therapy and how to control pain. I tell him my rule is to administer therapy as long as a patient responds well and has potential for a reasonably good quality of life, but that when all feasible therapies have been administered and a patient shows signs of rapid deterioration, I believe the continuation of therapy can cause more discomfort than cancer. I tell him I will then recommend surgery, radiotherapy, or chemotherapy only as a means of relieving pain. However, I assure him that if his condition should once again stabilize after the withdrawal of active therapy and if it should appear that he could still gain some good time, I will immediately reinstitute active therapy. I also assure each patient that there is an effective therapy to combat any degree of discomfort or pain and that I find the most effective procedure is simply to correlate the medication with the complaint. If he is nauseated, I will give him antinausea medicine. If he is unable to sleep, I will prescribe sedatives—barbiturate or nonbarbiturate, depending on his tolerance. And if he has pain, I will use an appropriate analgesic or narcotic, as often as needed. (These drugs can be administered in pill form, as a suppository, or by injection. A few patients even learn to administer their own shots, as a diabetic does, under medical supervision. Addiction is not a concern when a person has advanced cancer. Moreover, most patients report a tendency to use fewer drugs when they know drugs are readily available if needed.)

A patient has the right to give me instructions as to how he wants his last days handled. He can tell me where he wants to be and what he wishes in terms of medical support systems.

He may sign a "Directive to My Physician" form that will prohibit me or any other physician from giving him cardiac resuscitation or from using heroic measures to prolong his life.

(The question often arises as to whether a cancer patient who is acutely ill should be treated with cardiac resuscitation and/or intensive care. I believe a patient merits these procedures automatically if he or she has not yet undergone an adequate trial of anticancer therapy. Every effort should be made with each patient to strive for remission. However, I do not recommend a code blue and/or intensive care when a patient's disease has proved refractory to anticancer therapy and he is failing from advanced disease. The only exception I make to this policy is when a patient specifically requests that such procedures be implemented and when there is a remote possibility of success with additional therapy.)

Although the decision as to where he or she will die is the prerogative of each patient, this may be determined in part by practical considerations. Although most people would prefer to be at home, not every household can easily accommodate a patient who needs round-the-clock care. Other family members may be working, or they may be physically unable to carry out some of the more strenuous nursing duties such as turning the patient or helping him to the bathroom. The result of these and other factors is that today more people die in nursing homes and hospitals than at home. Dying in this manner, separated from familiar sights and sounds, can be a doubly lonely ordeal, increasing a person's natural feelings of isolation and abandonment. However, if I had to choose between these latter alternatives, I would recommend a hospital. Most nursing homes need to be upgraded before they can provide the medical facilities or the proper warmth and dignity for anyone, especially for the dying.

An ideal of care exists at St. Christopher's Hospice, in London. Founded by Dr. Cicely Saunders in 1967, St. Christopher's is a research, treatment, and teaching facility devoted to meeting the needs of the dying and the long-term sick. Its aims are both control of physical pain and understanding of the emotional and spiritual problems of such patients and their families. Dr. Saunders wants her patients to live until they die. The atmosphere is informal, the building designed for maximum openness, space, and light. Families are encouraged to visit at any hour of the day; and the staff becomes as friendly with them as with the patients. Children are welcome visitors. In such an atmosphere, a patient and his or her family can say a loving good-bye. It is a time of sadness but not of depression and emptiness. Similar hospices are now being founded in the United States.

Clearly, there are better and worse circumstances in which to die, and what I would call a *bad* death is one that occurs in the sterile atmosphere of a hospital or in the loneliness of a nursing home. A bad death is one where there is little communication between the dying person and his family or friends or the medical personnel, where there is no acknowledgment of the significance and sorrow to the patient of what is happening to him.

One of the best examples of a *good* death is that of Charles A. Lindbergh who died in August 1974. Diagnosed as having a lymphoma in 1972, he continued to live actively while undergoing radiotherapy and chemotherapy. He traveled extensively on conservation missions, which included promoting the preservation of a rare species of eagle and encouraging the study of the Stone Age Tasaday tribe in the Philippines. One of his doctors, Milton M. Howell, M.D.,[4] writes,

Chemotherapy was instituted and continued to the limit of its effectiveness.

From time to time, he returned to his beloved Kipahulu Valley, on the island of Maui, in Hawaii, a living museum of tropical foliage and wildlife. His contributions of time and effort had been considerable in preserving the area as a national park. Near this valley of a thousand waterfalls, he had personally helped clear the neglected graveyard beside the picturesque church built by Yankee missionaries. In time, he made appropriate legal arrangements for his burial there and selected the site of his grave. Systematically, he arranged his personal affairs, and yet he maintained a sense of the past and an interest in the present. He planned for the next major event of his life but it did not become an obsession.

As time passed, the inexorable progress of the disease forced his hospitalization in a major university center for several months. The best of medical efforts were made in his behalf; the finest of medical skills were applied. All this was insufficient to the task, for the neoplasm was the navigator of this flight.

Finally, in August 1974, a telephone call came to the village of Hana, Hawaii, from a hospital room in New York. "This is Charles Lindbergh. I have had a conference with my doctors, and they advise me that I have only a short time to live. Please find me a cottage or a cabin near the village. I am coming home to Maui." He did so. He was flown 5,000 miles on a litter.

He had made his decision, and he took full responsibility for it.

A cottage was found, overlooking the sea he loved. There, with two excellent nurses and his family, we participated along with him in the last eight days of his life.

He was elated for the first few days. His appetite improved. His fluid intake was adequate. There were regular morning conferences with the ranch superintendent to give instructions and receive reports on the progress of the construction of his grave and the building of his simple coffin. He planned his funeral service along with his family and requested that people attend in their work clothes. His days were full. There was time for reminiscing, time for discussion, and time for laughter. As his lungs filled, he required oxygen from time to time, and codeine, 15 mg as necessary. Finally, he lapsed into a coma and died twelve hours later. He wanted no respirator, defibrillator, or other complicated paraphernalia. None was available. He received excellent, prompt, responsive nursing care, oxygen when needed, a minimum of analgesia, and a great deal of love and consideration from his family and the medical staff.

He stated that he wished his death to be a constructive act in itself. His example of simplicity, his careful planning, his unfailing politeness and consideration for those around him, his public refusal of medical heroics, and his humble funeral are evidence of that wish. Death was another event in his life, as natural as his birth had been in Minnesota more than seventy-two years before.

Following the above article, Dr. Howell prints an excerpt from a letter written to him by Anne Morrow Lindbergh. It says, in part:

In the hospital in New York—excellent, thorough and tireless as the care was—there was always a veil between Charles and me, partly an inevitable physical veil because of the setup of a big hospital and routine . . . perhaps the veil was accidentally given by the doctors' and nurses' cheerful evasiveness . . . or perhaps due to my hesitancy in speaking first before Charles was ready to . . . and perhaps because Charles was trying to spare me from what I already knew . . . or perhaps he was not yet ready or able to broach such an emotional subject. Only in the last days there were we able to break through the veil, when Charles knew he was getting no better and he determined to go "home to Maui."

But it was the peace and beauty of Maui that we all could face together without fearing some of the fringes of its meaning. I am grateful for this opportunity to look at the mystery which everyone must meet in the end. For the boys it may have long-reaching effects down through their children and their children.

The death of Charles Lindbergh is an eloquent argument against the prolonged, futile use of advanced medical technology that sometimes results from a doctor's false optimism or unrealistic assessment of a patient's condition. In a manner similar to his, I am often asked by a patient to make funeral arrangements as well as assure that he or she not be given heroic measures when the end is near. The only thing a patient cannot dictate to me is when he will die, for there are no yardsticks to measure that delicate, highly individual time. Often I have seen a patient and thought that this was his time, only to find him so improved in the next few days that he returned home a week later. Therefore, I no longer feel that I or anyone else has the ability to predict when another person will die. I prefer to withhold judgment, visit a patient frequently, and continually reassess his condition.

When a patient goes into a final state of coma, however, I keep him comfortable by providing a moderate amount of hydration, frequent turning, and skin care. In certain cases I may continue to administer narcotics or sedatives at regular intervals if there appears to be restlessness or pain. This reassures his family that any pain or discomfort is being alleviated.

When death comes, it is not easy for a patient's family to accept, even when it means that the patient's suffering is over. At this time family members need special attention, which I try to provide along with other family members and friends, nurses, clergy, social workers, and hospital volunteers. I always hope that a family will find solace in the knowledge that its loved one has received good medical care and sensitive emotional support, that he lived as long and as well as possible under adverse conditions, and that all possible comfort was provided to ease his dying.

About ten days to two weeks after the death of a patient, the first flurry of attention from relatives and friends subsides, and the bereaved are alone with their despair. I try to help them by writing a letter in which I review the medical history of the patient, summarize his or her final days, and include any pertinent information obtained from the autopsy. I also discuss the important role played by the wife or husband or other family member in supporting the patient. Finally, I mention the normality of grieving and remind them that there will be a time when life will be less painful. I also invite them to visit me at any time if they feel I can help them with their problems of readjustment.

My goal, then, from the day I meet a patient until his cure, remission, or death, is to do everything I can to relieve the real and terrifying ordeal of living with cancer. Because I have witnessed it so often, I try to convince each patient that other people do live actively with disease; and I reassure him that if his disease is terminal, I can relieve his pain and suffering.

There is an understanding among people who work with

cancer patients and the patients themselves—something we all know and few of us ever learn—that it is not the length of a person's life that is important, but the quality of his days.

NOTES

1. Grace Halsell, "Mind over Cancer," *Prevention*, January 1976, pp. 118-127.
2. Arnon A. Fortgang, M.D., a surgeon in San Francisco, who planned to participate in the First National Training Conference for Physicians on "Psychosocial Care of the Dying Patient" by speaking of the patient's perspective on life-threatening illness, died on February 27, 1976.
3. John Hunt, "Life Before Death," *Proceedings of the Royal Society of Medicine*, 69:124, February 1976.
4. Milton M. Howell, "The Lone Eagle's Last Flight," *Journal of the American Medical Association*, 232(7):715-716, May 19, 1975.

PART II

THE RESPONSE OF THE HOSPICE

V

St. Christopher's Hospice

THELMA INGLES

The quality of care which dying patients receive, wherever they are—in hospitals, nursing homes, or their own homes— can be significantly influenced by nurses. However, this care must be given by nurses who are able to accept their own feelings about death, to listen compassionately and constructively to the fears of others, to provide both the physical and psychological support that enables patients to make the transition from life to death as peacefully as possible, and to support grieving families during the transition. It was at St. Christopher's Hospice in Sydenham, England that I came to know such nurses and began to appreciate that care given to the dying patient is a measure of man's humanity to man.

How can a dying patient be helped? And how can the family be supported during this time of grief and loss? I learned some answers during my three weeks as a volunteer staff nurse at St. Christopher's Hospice in Sydenham, England.

Most of all, I learned that the patient who is dying wants freedom from pain, yet not the dulling of awareness that interferes with his relationships with others. He wants friendliness and kindness and the comforting measures that tell him he is still important. He wants the familiar things that he

Thelma Ingles, former chairman of the graduate program of Duke University School of Nursing, has been advisor to many nursing programs, both in this country and in Latin America, and nursing consultant to the Rockefeller Foundation.

enjoyed when he was well—the favorite foods, flowers, music, the companionship of family and friends. He wants to be well groomed, attractively dressed. And, above all, he wants to be accepted as he is, to maintain his own individuality, and to be assured that when the time comes, he will be remembered with love and respect by those who have been close to him.

St. Christopher's comes as close to making these things possible as any place I have ever known. Unlike a hospital whose purpose is to treat sick people, a hospice is a place for dying. Its purpose is to help those patients who can no longer benefit from treatment to die as comfortably as possible, and to support their families and prepare them for the period of bereavement. At St. Christopher's, therefore, death is not seen as an academic subject—a phenomenon of interest to the pathologist, theologian, psychologist, anthropologist, or nurse. Instead it is seen as a very human event, a legitimate and normal process.

There is always time for kindness at St. Christopher's— "time in depth rather than length," as Dr. Cicely Saunders, its founder and guiding spirit, says. I remember the gentle kindness of the man who delivered the morning paper to the patients. He knew each patient by name, always had a few pleasant words to say, and was ready to make an extra effort to fulfill any unexpected request. One morning I said to him, "Do you know how much the patients love you?" He looked at me quietly for a moment and then said, "St. Christopher's does this to you, you know. Here there is always room for love."

And there is room for many other things as well. At St. Christopher's I never saw "last stand" measures used to prolong the dying process—no I.V.'s, no respirators, no emergency surgical procedures. Temperatures, pulse, respirations, and blood pressures are not taken. But great care is directed toward keeping patients comfortable—frequent changes of position, back rubs, tucked in pillows, bathing, good mouth care—attention to the small details that mean so much.

Furthermore, I never saw a patient suffer physically after the day of admission. Prevention of distressing symptoms is given the highest priority in the care schedule. Medications are dispensed on a schedule that keeps the patient comfortable—not held up until a patient must ask for relief. Heroin, permitted in England but not in this country, is often the drug of choice, because many physicians and nurses believe it has superior qualities over morphine. The use of both drugs and patients' responses to each is under study at St. Christopher's.

The wards of St. Christopher's are not gloomy places. You feel a pervasive tranquility, a peacefulness. There are always flowers on the patients' tables and plants in the windows. At the foot of each bed is a gay, handmade afghan. Every patient has earphones for TV and radio.

The nurses work in pairs—this facilitates lifting and moving patients, and permits a kind of interchange of support. There is often cheerful repartee between the patients and their nurses.

I remember one afternoon when a young Irish nurse brought a patient back to the ward. As they entered, the nurse began to sing and to dance around the patient—including her in the dance as much as possible. The other patients clapped the musical time. The patient looked shyly pleased, and a wave of good feeling spread through the ward.

Unlike most hospitals, St. Christopher's has few institutional rules. There is no age limit for visitors, and children are welcome. Once I remember seeing a woman surrounded by seven grandchildren whom she proudly introduced to me. Occasionally even the family dog is brought in for a visit. Visiting hours are unlimited except on Monday, which is known as "family day off"—the day when the patients don't expect a visit since they recognize that their families need a free day to do the normal things necessary in a home. Staff and volunteers plan special Monday activities—group sings, records, slides, talks, crafts, and so on—so the patients have no opportunity to feel lonely or neglected.

Furthermore, Monday was the day when my ward was transformed into a beauty salon—the day for shampoos, sets, and flattery. Looking well was important to the patients. The women especially wanted to look their best, and the nurses shared enthusiastically in the effort.

I remember a very sick patient who was given a permanent. Her previously lank, lifeless hair was suddenly converted into a mop of lovely white curls. She became the belle of the ward. That permanent meant a great deal to her—just the word itself was comforting.

In addition to looking well, the patients are interested in food. One of my frequent assignments was to carry the daily menu to the patients and mark their choices. Both for dinner and supper, they were able to choose between alternative entrees and desserts. This was important because it was one of the few opportunities for choices still available to them. Often they shared opinions on the relative merits of the alternatives.

Patients don't have to stop smoking; it is too late to try to change a life pattern. For some patients, smoking remains an enjoyable part of their daily routine, and it is not unusual to see patients smoke until a few hours before their death.

Cocktails are permitted, and families are encouraged to bring in the beverages that their relatives prefer. I remember one elderly woman who apologized to me each time she had her jigger of Scotch, apparently worried that I might have some puritanical scruples. So one afternoon, to ease her concern, I brought a highball to her bedside and we enjoyed our drinks together.

Most of the staff treated patients as individual, mature human beings. Only a few nurses occasionally lapsed into the paternalistic technique so common in hospitals where firm discipline is sometimes seen as essential to the success of a therapeutic regime. One patient's wife told me about a large London medical center where her husband had been a patient. "They treated him as if they owned him," she said, "and when I asked the nurses for information about his care, they saw me as an intruder. Patients in that hospital are a captive audience."

No one could call the patients at St. Christopher's captives. Their questions, and their families' questions, are answered honestly and with kindness. If a patient wants to talk about his disease or his prognosis, the nurse or the doctor finds time to sit down and talk with him. If a patient asks no questions, his right to privacy is respected and information is not imposed.

Sometimes a member of a patient's family, either because of a life pattern or out of the anxiety of the moment, becomes bossy: "Do this, don't do that." The staff is sensitive both to the anxiety which prompts the relative's behavior and to the patient's response to this treatment. For some patients, the behavior is simply a manifestation of the familiar; to others it demonstrates caring; and for others it is an irritation. If the latter, then time is planned for the family member to talk with one of the staff.

Almost all of the older patients are called by their family name—Mrs. Brown, Mr. Black, and the like. One exception was a ninety-two-year-old woman who was called "Mary," at her own request. For, as she told me, "I have no family—the nurses and doctors here are my family. *Mary* is more *family* than 'Miss Johnson.' " And so the staff said "Mary" as they would have said "dear," with affection rather than familiarity.

Religion is considered each individual's private affair. General prayers are said by a nurse each morning and evening, and most patients listen and participate. But an occasional patient "turns off" by reading or some other device, and this is perfectly acceptable, too.

One Sunday morning, I was asked to take the patients to chapel. I asked each person if he or she wanted to go and if the answer was yes, I took them—in bed, by wheelchair, on foot, or in whatever way we could manage.

I remember one choppy little woman, Mrs. Chalmers, on the Sunday she attended chapel for the first time. When the chaplain offered her the communion wafer, she said in a loud and convincing voice, "I don't want that thing." The chaplain moved quietly on to the next patient.

When we returned to the ward, she said to me, "Have you been confirmed?" When I replied "Yes," she said, "Well, I haven't been." I told her that because St. Christopher's has so few rules, I doubted that confirmation was required for communion.

Later I told the chaplain about my experience with Mrs. Chalmers. He said he would be glad to give her communion and, if she wished, he could arrange for her confirmation. He asked me to tell her for, as he put it, "If I go to her, she may feel I am pushing her. I wouldn't want this." Somehow, this attitude typifies St. Christopher's.

On another occasion, a thirty-four-year-old woman asked this same chaplain, "What will I do if the suffering becomes so great that I can't bear it?" He replied, "God won't ask more of you than you can bear." The patient felt such relief from his answer. He was right, too, because the nurses medicated her beyond the level of physical pain, and she went into a coma several hours before she died.

Whenever a patient dies, the curtains are drawn around the bed, and the nurses and family members present kneel around the bed as the head nurse reads prayers. I think this is helpful to the nurses, as well as to the relatives: it acknowledges the fact of death. After prayers, the patient is placed in as comfortable and peaceful position as possible and left in the bed, face uncovered, for one hour. Relatives can sit with the patient during this time, if they wish. If it seems appropriate, a nurse stays with the family.

At the end of the hour, the patient is removed to a private room, bathed, and taken in his bed to a small chapel where, if the family wishes, they can be joined by the chaplain or their own minister, priest, or rabbi. Thus, the family can remember the patient in his bed rather than in a satin-lined box. The body is then taken to a mortuary; cremation seems to be the choice in England.

As added comfort, families and friends of patients who have died in the hospice or under hospice care at home, are invited back to the "Pilgrim Club" to meet together one evening each month. Most of those who come are husbands or wives now left alone. They discuss their loneliness with one another and find solace in the sharing. This sharing of grief is an acceptable part of life at St. Christopher's. Some patients are able to express grief to the nurses and not to their families; for other patients, it's the other way around. But each one is helped to find his own way.

At St. Christopher's, I found that many dying patients became concerned about the way their relatives and friends would remember them. They wanted to be remembered for their strengths, not for their weaknesses. Most of all, they wanted to be remembered.

Many patients who are dying begin to review their relative strengths and weaknesses, their successes and their failures, their good behavior and bad behavior, the things they wish they had done, and the things they wish they had not done. The introspection may become painful, and some patients may need help in accepting themselves as they are and as they have been. Other patients may become suspicious and critical of their family, friends, and the staff, and need assistance in gaining a realistic perspective. To die peacefully, patients must be at ease with themselves and with others.

Trivial incidents may suddenly loom large and become burdensome. Patients may begin to contemplate the future, the meaning of death to themselves and to their families. Some patients may deny the possibility of death—it can't happen to me—and shy away from questions which might initiate the subject of death.

Their response to dying is influenced by so many factors—cultural background, philosophy of life, perception of themselves, their age, their relations with their families and friends, the value they place on life, the amount of suffering they can tolerate, and their religious faith. But, in whatever way each individual is able to come to grips with death, most patients need help with the dying process. The staff is alert to this need and is prepared to give the help that can make dying as tranquil as possible, both for the patients and their families.

The staff at St. Christopher's are continually helped to develop an attitude that enables them to comfort patients and families and to accept the reality that procedures which prolong the dying process are inappropriate and often cruel. In gaining this understanding they become freer in their approach to patients.

Inevitably, the relentless contact with grief is difficult for the staff. As a consequence, I sometimes saw manifestations of conflict, rudeness, and short tempers among the staff members, but I never saw this directed toward patients. This behavior struck me as a normal human reaction to the daily stress, and I believe the staff managed with remarkable control when one considers the tensions, anguish, and steady reminders of the impermanence of life with which they live.

Occasionally, of course, controls break down. When this happens, each member handles the situation in his or her own way—crying, display of anger, keeping especially busy, going to chapel, drinking coffee, talking with friends, or just sitting quietly with a selected patient.

Understandably, the staff, as well as the patients, are constantly in need of support. This is provided on a regular basis at ward meetings and routine group conferences. When the leadership of these conferences is good, they are very useful. The chaplain and the chief tutor were particularly sensitive to the reactions of individuals and able to give the kind of support which leads to useful insight.

St. Christopher's care is not limited to the patients under its roof. Its home care program, associated with its clinic, includes some persons not yet admitted to the hospice, as well as others who have been discharged—for a while, at least. The nurses in the program work with the district nurses and general practitioners.

The drug schedule for home patients is planned by the St. Christopher's staff, and the hospice nurses make periodic home visits to monitor drug schedules and support patients and families. A nurse is always on call twenty-four hours a day so the families are sure of getting help whenever they need it.

The certainty of being able to talk with someone they know gives the family confidence, and they do not abuse the system. If a nurse receives a call at night, she may be able to handle the situation on the phone or may make a home visit there and then. It's her decision.

I was impressed by the way patients and families responded to the nurses. One patient said to me, "I feel so safe when the nurse comes. It's as if I have a back-up team behind me; I don't have to be scared."

Sometimes when a family seems extremely tired, the nurse may suggest that the patient be admitted to St. Christopher's for a while so that the family can get some rest. I remember visiting one home where the patient was in the last stages of his illness and his wife was exhausted. The nurse did not abruptly recommend the hospice, but rather led up to it as a possibility for the near future. Several days later, by mutual agreement between husband and wife, the patient was admitted.

Approximately 10 percent of the hospice patients go home for periods of time once their symptoms are controlled. They are followed closely by the clinic nurses. At holiday times patients often are taken home, by car or ambulance, for several days.

Patients on home care have regular scheduled clinic visits as long as they are able to travel, and the clinic routine at St. Christopher's is in marked contrast to that seen in most other places. At St. Christopher's, patients are not kept waiting. The schedule is carefully planned so that each patient can be given optimum care. There is time to answer the patient's and family's questions, and the home care routine is modified according to the current symptoms. After the clinic visit, the patients and their spouses (or other family members) are invited to have lunch in the dining room.

They may be joined there by some of the volunteers who are attracted to work at St. Christopher's; some are wives or husbands of patients who have died at St. Christopher's or elsewhere. These patients make excellent helpers because they understand the problems of the patients and families; they've been through it themselves. At the same time, serving as volunteers helps them to work out the loneliness of their own loss.

Some of the volunteers are nurses who give one day or a half day a week of service. Other volunteers work hard and provide many small but important services. They take care of flowers, carry trays, feed patients, wash patients' soiled laundry, assist with nursing care, run errands for patients and staff, make phone calls to families, sit with patients, or participate in recreational therapy.

No job seems too dirty or too hard for the volunteers because they are truly motivated with the spirit of good will. I have never seen volunteers contribute as much to the service of a ward as those volunteers at St. Christopher's do. It is possible that the volunteers who have had a recent bereavement need to keep busy and feel useful, but all the volunteers seem to possess a natural courtesy and the capacity for love. That is probably why they choose to help at St. Christopher's—and why they add so much to the care there.

Today, with the great emphasis on prolonging life, whatever its meaning, the nurse may enter a patient's room only to give a useless injection, to monitor ineffectual equipment, to count the drops of intravenous solution, to check the suction apparatus, or to measure drainage. None of these activities requires the nurse to touch the patient or to speak to him. Indeed, nurses may find little time to *see* the person in the bed or to *hear* the questions of the worried family. Things seem to have taken precedence over people, efficiency over caring.

No one questions the appropriate use of miracle drugs or life-saving equipment; the point is that nurses must not see them as substitutes for caring. The secret of the care of patients is still caring. This is particularly true in the care of dying patients; there may be little else really valid to offer. Although a patient and his family may wish desperately for life to continue, prolongation of the dying process may be an intensely destructive ordeal for both. To temper the process, kindness must be "as large and plain as a prairie wind." The staff at St. Christopher's understand this concept and put it into practice daily.

VI

Hospices for the Dying, Relief from Pain and Fear

CONSTANCE HOLDEN

This country is pouring millions of dollars into the war against cancer, but is not paying much heed to the plight of victims once their individual battles are lost.

Of the 700,000 people diagnosed as having cancer each year, two out of three die of their malignancies. For these people dying can be a slow, painful, and very lonely business. Hospitals, geared as they are to aggressive therapy and prolongation of life, do not offer a good milieu for dying. A person is not necessarily better off at home if he is alone or surrounded by an anxious, grieving family, ill-prepared to give him proper care.

Despite the growing concern about death and dying in this country, there is not much understanding of the needs of dying people—the needs for comfort both physical and mental, for others to see them as individuals rather than as hosts of their diseases, for someone to breach the loneliness and help them come to terms with the end.

Hospices—homes for care of the dying—are one way to meet the problem. The hospice idea, which originated among religious orders in the Middle Ages, has its modern flowering in England where a number of such places have been set up for attending to dying cancer patients. These differ from the

Constance Holden is a staff writer for Science, *a publication of the American Association for the Advancement of Science.*

"Hospices for the Dying, Relief from Pain and Fear," Holden, C., *Science*, Vol. 193, pp. 389-391, 30 July 1976. Copyright 1976 by the American Association for the Advancement of Science.

kind that are still run by charitable religious groups in one significant respect: in addition to loving concern for patients they are undergirded by a solid medical component whose chief characteristic is the sophisticated management of severe pain and other unpleasant symptoms of terminal cancer.

Best known to professionals in this country is St. Christopher's Hospice in London, founded less than a decade ago by Dr. Cicely Saunders. The hospice, which also does some pharmacological and psychosocial research, has become something of a mecca for health professionals interested in terminal care, which Saunders calls a "largely unexplored medical field." Not only is it novel to the high-technology big-business system of medical care we have, but it embodies a rather rare combination of spirituality and hard medicine, a combination whose uniqueness may not be appreciated until one encounters it in such a person as Cicely Saunders.

Saunders, now in her mid-fifties, is an Oxford-educated (philosophy, politics, economics) lady who broke off her studies to become a nurse during World War II. An injured back sent her back to university where she finished her degree and became a medical social worker. Her hospice idea was born during the course of a close friendship with a forty-year-old Polish refugee who was dying of cancer in a busy London hospital. They discussed the kind of place where he would like to be, and he left her £500 when he died to help set up her "Home." Saunders went on to get her medical degree and subsequently spent seven years at St. Joseph's, a London hospice. Finally, in the late 1960's, she received money from the National Health Service to build St. Christopher's, a five-story building in southeast London.

Saunders' unique contribution to hospices has been the sound medical management of terminal cancer pain. The first goal at St. Christopher's is to make the patient free of pain, and of the memory and fear of pain, by arranging that continuous dosages of analgesics be given so the patient is always one step ahead of the pain. In the most severe cases, this means regular oral doses of what is know as the Brompton mix, a cocktail made up of diamorphine (heroin), cocaine, gin, sugar syrup, and chlorpromazine syrup. The diamorphine dose starts at 5 to 10 milligrams, and patients rarely need more than 30 milligrams at a time. Saunders explains that when a patient's fears and anxieties are relieved the dosages can often be lowered, because so much of the subjective sensation of pain comes from emotional distress.

Sophisticated use of analgesics is a hallmark of St. Christopher's—indeed, says Saunders, "better pain control in hospitals would make many admissions [to the hospice] unnecessary." Inadequate pain control in hospitals is attributable partly to pharmacological ignorance on the part of doctors, and partly to the belief that analgesics should be administered sparingly to prevent the patient from becoming addicted and to avoid damaging side effects. But such considerations are irrelevant to the dying. When the principles of pain control for a patient who is expected to get well are applied to the terminally ill, the results are often appallingly inhumane.

At St. Christopher's, there is no such thing as giving "too much" analgesic—there is only that which is sufficient for continuous pain control. Saunders says this is not achieved at the expense of turning a patient into an insensate zombie. Further, she claims, a patient, once made comfortable, never develops a psychological addiction to the opiates.

Pain control is only part of what makes the hospice unusual. The rest comes from the atmosphere created by constant attention by the staff and volunteers who spend much time just listening and hand-holding (there is much more physical contact than in hospitals), and by the presence of friends and family members who can drop by almost any time and sometimes spend the whole day at the patient's bedside.

Saunders arrived at the NIH Clinical Center one day to explain her hospice, with the aid of a collection of slides. She resembles the stereotype of a typical English matron, tall and generously bosomed, but the moment she began to speak one could understand why one American doctor calls her a "startlingly beautiful woman." She radiates vitality, intelligence, and joyous humor. She is also a serious Christian.

Saunders explained that the character of the hospice has a lot to do with the community where it is located, a close-knit neighborhood in southeast London. Patients—those with the worst pain get first priority—are drawn from a 6-mile radius containing 1.5 million people. The hospice has seventy beds, fifty-four for cancer patients—average length of stay is twelve days—and a sixteen-bed wing for frail elderly patients, some of whom are relatives of staff members. Patients are in four-bed bays so they are never alone. There is sun and fresh flowers, and patients are surrounded by photographs and other personal belongings. Visiting hours are 8 a.m. to 8 p.m., and relatives are all over the place. Saunders showed several "before" and "after" slides of patients on admission—their faces and bodies showing tension and fear—and several days afterwards—one man, for example, had lost his hollow-eyed look and was propped up in bed, reading the racing form. She showed a man several days before his death, his face half eaten away by cancer, surrounded by friends and cheerily lifting a glass of sherry to celebrate his birthday. ("Celebration is a very important part of terminal care.") One man "died in his chair by his bed with his glasses on, which is how we want him to be," said Saunders cheerfully. Some patients can go home for a while after their pain is brought under control, bringing their Brompton mix with them in a big blue bottle. One such woman, a victim of stomach cancer, was shown working in the kitchen, her small children at her knees, two weeks before her death. The hospice people know that children can cope with death much better when the dying relative is not stashed away, a fact poignantly illustrated by a picture of a child reading a comic book next to the bed of his dying father.

Children, of course, are good to have around, and there is a nursery for offspring of the staff on the grounds of the hospice. Families are encouraged to help with patients' care. When someone dies, the staff mourns too. Relatives are looked after to see how they handle bereavement and those thought to be "at risk" are visited frequently by staff members and volunteers. Monthly parties are held for families and staff members.

Saunders emphasizes that medical care at St. Christopher's is "appropriate" care—which is to say, it is the patient and not the disease that gets the attention. She showed a picture of a new patient who came in with tubes sticking out of him from a tracheostomy and a gastrostomy. This, she said, was not "appropriate"; while it may have removed some of the tumor, it did nothing for the person.

The English are not very big on psychiatry, tending more toward reliance on common sense. A psychiatrist does sit in on the frequent staff meetings to help participants communicate with each other and to offer advice on dealing with patients in particular emotional distress. It may well be asked how the staff can handle such constant association with death. Some can't take it but most can; as Saunders says, what they are seeing is "not constant pain, but constant relief of pain." Of course, it takes some optimism and serenity to see this last phase as Saunders does: as "the unique period in the patient's illness when the long defeat of living can be gradually converted into a positive achievement in dying."

The hospice is not cheap to run—the per patient cost is about 80 percent of that in a general hospital in England—and 85 percent of the budget goes to staff salaries. "We are high person, low technology and hardware," says Saunders. But there are more savings over hospital care than these figures imply, because they do not take into account the fact that the home care program enables many people to die at home who would otherwise be in the hospital.

Whereas in the past some members of the medical establishment have tended to regard people like Saunders as pious eccentrics, the hospice idea now appears to be catching on in England, where twenty-two additional hospices are now being planned.

But it is hard to predict how successfully the concept could be incorporated into the American health care system. There are many variables that will determine whether such places can avoid taking on the grim aura of nursing homes or developing a creepy reputation as places where people go to die. Keeping the place alive, and not a "cul-de-sac," in Saunders' phrase, requires full community and family involvement.

Some American doctors are cautious about the hospice idea. John C. Hisserich of the Cancer Center at the University of Southern California is eager to see the idea tried, but he warns that no scientific evaluation has been made of hospice care and that the evidence of success is largely anecdotal. He also believes that hospice enthusiasts sometimes exhibit "a certain zealotry about the thing that may be necessary but that has the effect of turning off physicians who might otherwise be interested. . . ."

Perhaps the most serious reservations about efforts to sprout hospices in America come from Mel Krant, director of cancer programs at the new University of Massachusetts School of Medicine in Worcester. "My first reaction," he says, "is it's going to fail as an American idea. It will get into operation but its intent will fail." The reason, he feels, is that hospices will simply add to the excessive fragmentation, over-specialization, and discontinuity in American medicine. A hospice will be the incarnation of yet another specialty—care of the dying—and will become "another discontinuous phenomenon" when what is needed is integration. Krant has high regard for the English hospices, but he fears that without the spirit of voluntarism and community feeling that exists in England, and without leaders as "utterly devoted" as Cicely Saunders, hospices will turn out looking like nursing homes. He also thinks hospices would help relieve hospitals and physicians of their true responsibilities, which should include more community involvement. Krant thinks it better that Americans develop their own indigenous models for incorporating hospice concepts.

While others are more optimistic than Krant, there is wide agreement that ideally there should be a limited need for special facilities to take care of the dying because, with adequate education and technical and emotional support, the majority of patients who die in hospitals could be seen through the end at home. Adds another physician, "If we're going to solve the problem of terminal patients, an increasing number of patients will have to die in the bosom of their own home." (How many is open to question. What of all the old people who have no family into whose bosom they may retreat?)

This will take some attitude-changing, not only among the general populace, but among members of the medical profession who find it difficult to get out of what Saunders calls the "investigate-diagnose-prolong-cure" mode of treatment and to redirect their energies to bringing relief from pain and isolation. The way things are conducted at the English hospices seems strange to doctors who have been trained as therapeutic activists—one doctor, after two months at St. Christopher's, wrote that he was struck by the absence of temperature, pulse, and blood pressure rounds and by the fact almost no intravenous fluids were given or blood samples taken. It was "a contradiction to all my previous training. And sometimes my inability to cure a patient became almost unbearable." Finally he found new kinds of satisfactions—"from helping to transform a patient in severe pain into one pain-free and at peace."

A sidelight, but perhaps a very significant one, to the hospice philosophy bears on its relationship to the euthanasia controversy. Richard Lamerton, the young medical officer at St. Joseph's Hospice who has written and lectured in the field, writes: "If anyone really wants euthanasia, he must have pretty poor doctors and nurses." For, he says, when concern for the patient's well-being replaces dogged attacks on a disease that is hopelessly out of control, the euthanasia dilemma ceases to exist. In hospices, for example, patients are not fed intravenously if they want to stop eating. Antibiotics are not automatically given for the pneumonia of a terminal patient. When an ulcerated artery begins hemorrhaging, the patient is not given transfusions when the end is clearly in sight anyway; instead he is covered with a blanket so he won't be frightened at the sight of his blood and administered a strong sedative while someone sits close by clasping his hand. To Lamerton, this is not "passive euthanasia" but "appropriate care."

Such procedures do not mean that a patient couldn't be given aggressive life-prolonging therapy until the end if he wanted it. The hospice movement does not represent a new approach toward dying, but simply an attempt to establish as standard those principles that have always guided the best practitioners.

VII
Reflections of a Hospice Chaplain
THE REV. PAUL S. DAWSON

The following reflections are presented not as an exhaustive picture of hospice chaplaincy, but as a collection of insights from my own experience in this fascinating ministry. Each dying patient and his family and close circle of friends are unique and special. Each relationship in hospice calls the chaplain to a new frontier, a new adventure toward understanding human living and dying. It is mainly for this reason that I have outlined general conditions, none of which is foreign to the ordinary life experience. The difference is that with the dying and those closest to them, these conditions are unavoidable and increasingly insistent. They demand a reckoning if one is to have a good death. Insofar as hospice care raises the quality of life of the terminal patient to a high level, the responsibility of the hospice care staff to attend to the spiritual requirements of the patient and his loved ones is correspondingly heightened. Of all members of the team, the chaplain must uphold this spiritual responsibility. I hope that this brief essay will help readers in meeting that awesome challenge—awesome because it is immersed in the terrible mysteries of life at its fullest, and of death approached consciously, deliberately, and courageously.

The hospice chaplain is continuously faced with questions that seem to defy answers. The pressure to supply answers is sometimes enormous. It is soon apparent that in the face of death, certain questions are unavoidable and unan-

---

The Reverend Paul S. Dawson is presently an Episcopal Chaplain at the Church Home and Hospital in Baltimore, Maryland.

swerable in rational terms. We can learn to live with them, cope with them, and hopefully transcend them, but these questions remain open and profoundly provocative nonetheless. We cannot be God, nor must we play God—but we can in priestly fashion represent him to those who look to us for help, and we can offer them to Him at the throne of divine grace. Sometimes that is all we can do, and having done it, we must let go and go about our work.

There are times when we shall do badly and make costly and irreversible mistakes, and these mistakes will be all the more horrifying because time is so short, and we want to save the day, not lose it. At these times especially we must not play God—but we can, hopefully, learn from our mistakes. At such low times a cohesive, caring, and nourishing staff can compensate for our inadequacies and can help promote healing and growth in us. It is helpful then to remember the miracles that are worked through this remarkable form of creative care in an area that until recently has been grievously neglected and shrouded in the darkness of ignorance and fear. Behind my reflections is the expectation that each of us has the wherewithal to die well, as each of us, given the chance and the will, has the wherewithal to live well.

Personal fulfillment requires that we accept and work within our individual milieu and language. At its deepest level, that milieu and language can be private, protected, inchoate, and/or unconscious. Hospice work occurs against the background of our own existence and those to whom we relate— a background which ultimately opens out against the infinite reaches of eternity. The process of ministering to the dying and those closest to them becomes, then, a shared pilgrimage in which we learn from one another, nourish one another, experience intimacy, and stand as one before the primal mysteries of life, suffering, and death. With Donne we would surely agree that each man's death diminishes us. Yet it is also true that successful communion with our brothers and sisters and the "one God and Father of all, who is over all and through all and in all," gives us the power to grow and experience the true nobility of the human condition. The language of engagement and sharing at this level is more often non-verbal and mythopoeic than logical and concrete. The goal is the person-to-person communion between men and with God of which Tournier speaks.[1] There is no escape from the essential questions, nor are they dissipated with much rhetoric (though Christ "overcame" suffering and death once and for all, we still must suffer and die—but we know that in Christ we will not be overwhelmed). One comes to terms with the essential questions by the discovery of a new perspective, a new condition for living which admits the difficult questions rather than denying them.

In the Pulitzer Prize-winning play *The Shadow Box* we find examples of some basic questions that plague the dying and their loved ones. The three leading characters are dying, and they are each surrounded by loved ones.

Brian, while talking to his ex-wife who has come to visit and his male lover with whom he is presently living, says:

> And I'm just as alive as I ever was. And I *will* be alive right up to the last moment. *That's* the hard part, that last fraction of a second—when you know that the next fraction of a second—I can't seem to fit that moment into my life . . . You're absolutely alone facing an absolute unknown and there is absolutely nothing you can do about it . . . except give in.[2]

Brian seems to be saying: I am present and alive right now— I know it and feel it, and those closest to me know it and feel it, but will there be a live presence when I die? If so, where and how will I be present, and with whom? *What's going to happen to me?*

While reminiscing about the events and experiences of the past, and the hopes and dreams for the future, Joe, another character, says to his wife and teen-age son:

> So many goddam things. Where do they go? The freezer, the washer and the dryer, a dishwasher for Christ's sake, the lawn mower, the barbecue, three bicycles, four, six lawn chairs and a chaise lounge—aluminum, last forever—the white table with the umbrella, the hammock, the bar, I put that wood paneling in the basement, we

finished the attic—well, half of it, I got the insulation in—the patio, with screens . . . Jesus, it was a lot to let go of.[3]

What does it all matter? Life goes on all around me, Joe is saying, but what about my life—our life—all that we accumulated, all that we are, all that we hope for and yearn to become?

Agnes, whose mother is dying, is discussing with an interviewer her decision to deceive her mother into thinking her dead sister is alive. Agnes began writing letters to her mother from that sister, weaving a life-story that is fictional, but which supports her mother in a way that Agnes cannot:

It means so much to her. It's important to her. It's something to hope for. You have to have something. People *need* something to keep them going.[4]

What does it all mean—what's the use—who cares? Such questions are recurring themes in the world of the dying. They are never entirely resolved, they never quite disappear—they come to haunt when the going gets rough. They point up several basic needs—or conditions which are perennially human, and particularly urgent at this time.

INTIMACY

To a great extent, our own sense of well-being and personal identity depends upon the regard in which we are held by those closest to us. Many of the elderly hospice patients have a very small circle of friends and/or family, if any at all. The imperative atmosphere in which the dying find themselves brings conflicts and problems out into the open, particularly where feelings are concerned. This is especially difficult for patients who have been brought up and have remained in a climate in which a display of affection and closeness has been discouraged. Others may pride themselves on an attitude of independence and self-sufficiency, so that in their last days it is difficult for them to be dependent gracefully or to form close ties with anyone. But in all terminal patients the need for intimacy is strong, however hidden, and however difficult it may be to express feelings. These patients need the support and reinforcement that intimacy provides because they can actually see and feel life slipping away. Dying often brings a person to a state of great dependence and vulnerability. The high priority placed on caring in hospice programs helps to meet this need, but the chaplain, in relating to the patient as God's representative, is able to establish a closeness that speaks for eternity as well as for the present moment. The chaplain's familiarity with the "things of God"—Scripture, prayer, the sacraments—equips him or her with the ability to represent God in a uniquely focused and intense way. The chaplain can help to interpret what is happening in the light of its religious implications (remembering that the patient presents symbols—sometimes in dreams or in visions—and it is the patient, ultimately, who must read them and feel comfortable with their interpretation). The chaplain must be very cautious not to impose, however implicitly, prejudices on his caring approach to the patient. I feel strongly that it is an uncharitable and self-righteous person who takes advantage of another's vulnerability and need in order to convert or bully him into a different frame of mind. True loving care accepts the person where and as he or she is—if there is a change, it will come through example, and the person will gesture for guidance or information. I have found that trusting the regenerative power of intimacy itself to bring about whatever change is appropriate is far the better way. Of course, one must be sensitive to the implications in shy gestures and awkward or clumsy expressions. We all communicate simultaneously at several levels; for example, an angry response may veil fear or panic, or a sense of abandonment. An attitude of patient, listening kindness can touch the person behind his defenses. The realization that one is understood in spite of barriers and facades provides groundwork for an intimate relationship where it is desperately needed.

I have often noticed how loved ones and staff tend to withdraw from the dying person, particularly as debilitating symptoms become more evident. The dying person is treated as though he were already dead; he is seen merely as an object or an unresponsive and perhaps repulsive "thing." What a difference when this wasted "thing's" personhood is recognized, respected, and loved; when his right to live fully is recognized, acknowledged, and reinforced by those closest to him; when his history is reviewed and shared by those who are most involved in it; when he is affirmed as a valuable and meaningful person through an environment distinguished as a community of love.

Emotional and physical expressions of affection are indispensable for intimacy. With them, one realizes that his life is incorporated into the lives of those who mean most to him. Laying-on-of-hands, whether or not with spoken prayer, is helpful and strengthening. One of the glories of hospice care is the symptom control that ensures the highest quality of life for the dying, often enabling patients to return home to become a functioning part of their families and communities. But it is cruel to enable a person to live fully if we are not at the same time prepared to be equally open if that is needed. I have seen many instances of "a new lease on life" emerging in the dying patient as death looms close and becomes unavoidable—one of the many paradoxes that underscores the creative and now-or-never character of hospice care.

One is filled with awe, as in the presence of holiness, when one beholds the radiancy that is so evident in a person who is "dying well." It's as though the spiritual body is free to glow with a minimum of encumbrance when the physical body fades and dissolves. This "glorious" presence is clearly indestructible and a reproach to our frightened clutch on mortal life.

Intimacy enables one to share negative as well as positive experiences and facets of the personality. A "conspiracy of silence" in the world of the dying springs from a desire to spare feelings, or to avoid dealing with feelings that may be negative or ugly (e.g., guilt, grief, resentment, and anger). Intimacy involves a willingness to enter into another's pain and "shadow" side, and a willingness to share our own pain, insecurities, and "shadow" side.[5] When one shares intimately with the dying, one "walks through the valley of the shadow of death." But one also walks as a pioneer into the virgin country of new life and vibrant hope, where unexpected discoveries and insights carry their own nourishment and reward.

POVERTY

Intimacy with the dying and those close to them inevitably brings us to a confrontation with impoverishment; impoverishment which comes from recognizing the foolishness, impotence, and mortality of any one creature's life reflected against the vastness of the universe. We can only bear, at any stage in life, to see a little of this poverty that distinguishes human life. The dying, however, are immersed in it—the signs of their creatureliness and finiteness surround them on every side, as they sink into the commonness of death. It must be accepted, and it can be more readily accepted if those closest to the patient can share their own impoverishment. Hospice care provides a laboratory by which we can accept our impoverished selves through this kind of sharing, and in doing so, can open the door to wholeness for ourselves. None of us can be healed or made whole when we refuse to acknowledge the negatives and the poverty of our own existence. Coming to terms with this side of ourselves helps to defuse the *hubris* (the drive in all of us to displace God and establish absolute and invincible security for ourselves) that makes humility impossible. "Blessed are ye poor, for yours is the kingdom of God" (Luke 6:20; or as the New English Bible so aptly states in Matthew: "How blest are those who know their need of God; the kingdom of Heaven is theirs"). The example of Jesus Christ's poverty, his acceptance of it, and its paradoxical significance in his role as Savior, speaks for itself.

LETTING GO

It is hard to let go of what we do not ultimately own. Another way of putting this is that we cling more desperately to something of value when it is being taken from us, when our hold is no longer totally secure. In the deepest sense, our lives are not our own—so much happens to us quite apart from our own control. Our life history is viewed more vividly when we are dying, because it is through our history that we orient ourselves and find the pattern for the security we seek. The present moment is an impingement of the past and future onto the now. So long as death is a remote possibility, we can plan to rectify or resolve the past and look for fulfillment in the future. But of course the past and future are dead except they are given life by the present. People who are dying relive their history daily, as though, in slow motion, their lives were flashing before their eyes. They have a need for recapitulation, for reviewing their past in order to redeem it, to make sense out of it, to claim it as their own. The importance of healing memories is apparent.[6]

I am not convinced that every dying person requires an open-ended future. I have known persons who have faced death calmly with the firm conviction that "it all ends there." But for most, recapitulation emerges as a threshold for a new beginning, transcending the past without losing its essential meaning. In order for this to occur, detachment is required, a gradual letting-go of one's past in order to be able to leap out into a "larger life."

Guilt from remorse at the failure of love and responsibility with regard to self, others, and God represents a serious obstacle to such detachment. The minister can act as an agent of reconciliation in broken and torn families, helping to bring about understanding where reconciliation is impossible.

What cannot be changed can be accepted through a new way of looking at an old problem, an old hurt, an unresolved conflict. Each step in the detachment or letting-go process is a death in itself, making the final release easier. Where guilt is concerned, absolution can come only from God, and the chaplain can be the channel for such absolution, either formally through Confession and Absolution, or in Protestant ministries by listening and giving prayerful assurance of pardon. Where this ministry is not possible, communication, at least, can be improved and sometimes restitution can be made. Where there has been a failure of love and responsibility, healing comes through a restoration of love and a resurgence of response. Hospice care aims at healing broken families, and reestablishing lines of communication and responsibility where that is possible. I have seen many instances where this has happened against all odds. The peace that comes to the dying person when such efforts do work has an almost miraculous effect in making death easier.

Letting-go makes way for healing and integration—an empty vessel is ready to be filled—a soul, trim and reduced to essentials, is prepared for the unknown. "If a man has faith in me, even though he die, he shall come to life; and no one who is alive and has faith shall ever die" (John 11:26).

MEANING

Meaning comes from a sense of being valued in oneself, and of being needed. It comes also from awareness of being part of a whole larger than oneself. The stress in hospice care upon the family as part of the patient's world affects the work of the chaplain as mediator and minister of reconciliation. Where the patient is an active member of a church, the community of the faithful has a special importance, thus emphasizing the role of the minister as the head of the parish family.

Meaning which stretches beyond one's own finitude and upholds it has a mythic nature, and as it comes into awareness, it is often marked by symbols that appear in dreams, fantasies, and visions. These often have a very beautiful significance, but sometimes seem almost banal to any but the dying person. I recall one lady in middle age whose sense of underlying meaning was symbolized in a series of dreams and visions. For example, at one point in her last hospitalization, a huge mansion appeared before her hospital bed at the same time every evening. She was invited to enter, and spent much time wandering through its halls and rooms in wonder and expectation. She always returned after such a visit, realizing that her time had not yet come but she knew that before long, this beautiful place would be her home. On one occasion, a great boat on a limitless sea appeared instead of the house, and a skiff was rowed to the shore to pick her up and carry her aboard the vessel, where she saw the variety of animals and forms of life in pairs that identified it as Noah's ark. She was asked by Noah if she would like to travel with them to the distant shore, but realizing again that it was not time for her to leave, she returned to shore—and it was just a week or so after that incident that she died. I was continuously charmed and in awe of these visions as she related them to me, and felt very privileged to be asked to share them with her (she apparently discussed them with no one else). As death drew near, this lady, who had before her illness become estranged from her family and her church, experienced reconciliation with her family and with God, receiving the full sacramental ministry—and this brought an ever increasing sense of peace and resolution. The power that shone from her presence as she neared death was humbling to those who ministered to her at the end. This sense of meaning, when it occurs, takes on the character of a metamorphosis, evolving through a series of transitions from one form of life or living to another. Occasionally patients experience frightening visions in which those closest to them, including the chaplain, take on a threatening or demonic mien. The experience can be so real and convincing that no amount of explanation suffices to uproot it. This can be attributed to "organic psychosis" brought on by metastasis to the brain, sensory deprivation, drugs, or lack of sufficient nourishment. Even so, the symbols which emerge in such "bad trips" are sometimes related to the spiritual metamorphosis which is in progress at a deeper level.

The chaplain in a hospice program inevitably becomes involved in the needs of the staff. This is a two-way process, since spiritual ministry is the responsibility of all staff members, and is by no means the exclusive province of the clergy. The threat of "burn-out" is always present for all members of the interdisciplinary team. Emotional concentration is so intense and the pressures to be responsive so constant that sensitive monitoring of the emotional climate and the provision of healthy outlet and opportunity for change of pace are vital to a healthy hospice process. All the arts that are brought to bear in relating to patients and their loved ones must be available as well for the staff. The chaplain must have the grace to receive such ministry from those with whom he works so closely.

Finally, we are brought to see again that the questions

raised by terminal illness are profound and open-ended—the kinds of questions relating to existence, suffering, and death that have plagued philosophers, theologians, and poets for as long as culture has existed. We cannot hope to be ready with answers for such questions, but we can offer a faithful presence, a caring heart, a listening ear, a discerning intelligence, and the eternal graces available in the fellowship of the Spirit, prayer, Scripture, and the sacraments.

cc. 30Nov80e
(H+c)   The best thing that we can do is to bring to the hospice ministry the best that we are. If our ministry rests on a sure faith in a loving and caring God, this will come through in our sharing with the patients, families, and staff. To the same extent that we let our lives rest in the providence of God, so we carry the lives of others to the throne of grace. A sound life in God is its own best witness for Him. The centering in God in such a life is infectious, and its graces brim over to affect the lives it touches.

NOTES

1. Paul Tournier, *The Meaning of Persons* (New York: Harper & Row, 1975).
2. Michael Cristofer, *The Shadow Box* (New York: Samuel French, Inc., 1977), p. 43.
3. *Ibid.*, pp. 67, 68.
4. *Ibid.*, p. 60.
5. Henri J. M. Nouwen, *Out of Solitude* (Indiana: Ave Maria Press, 1966). There is a particularly fine and beautiful exposition of the word "care" in this little book, in which the author indicates that caring for another involves entering into his suffering with a willingness to share its burdens intimately.
6. Dennis and Matthew Linn, *Healing of Memories* (New York: Paulist Press, 1974). This book develops the idea, first suggested by Agnes Sanford, of submitting crippling memories to the healing power of the Holy Spirit—a positive act of offering them to God. The authors commend the Sacrament of Absolution as a particularly effective way of doing this.

VIII
Pain Control in Terminal Illness
SYLVIA A. LACK, M.B., B.S.

PRINCIPLES OF PAIN CONTROL

The patient with a diagnosis of cancer frequently waits in a misery of apprehension for the pain to start. The physician needs to be aware that as many as 50 percent of cancer patients do not suffer pain during the course of their illness. Of the remaining 50 percent, another 10 percent have only mild pain, leaving 40 percent with moderate to severe pain.[1] So much can be done to alleviate pain that the physician is justified in optimism and determination to control the pain of terminal cancer.

These facts about the pain associated with cancer should be conveyed to the patient very early in the course of the disease. Although the physician has been unable to control the disease process itself, causing frustration to both physician and patient, a valid base of trust can be established and maintained in the area of pain control. The first mild pain should be taken seriously and controlled adequately, thereby establishing confidence that the physician does have skills to prevent discomfort. This confidence will be a powerful ally if pain does become a troublesome problem later in the illness.

Effective pain control is based upon a tripod of treatment supporting the primary goal: a pain-free patient with normal affect. Mental acuity need not be sacrificed to the cause of

Dr. Sylvia Lack worked for two years at St. Christopher's and St. Joseph's Hospice in London before coming to this country to help establish The Connecticut Hospice, Inc. in New Haven, of which she is presently Medical Director.

freedom from pain; pain need not be the price paid for awareness. The patient can be alert to friends, family and surroundings without drug-induced drowsiness or euphoria and yet be
without pain. A normal mental state can be sustained through
a three-faceted approach. The physician must consider (1)
identification of the pain's source, (2) continuous pain relief
and (3) ease of administration.

Identification of the pain's etiology, the medical term for
source, is important since cancer does not preclude other ills;
simultaneous non-malignant sources of pain must also be
considered. Cystitis, hemorrhoids, toothache and angina may
require specific remedies. The cause of pain should be primarily a clinical diagnosis. Extensive investigations are not
usually appropriate or necessary for the terminally ill. They
should be non-invasive and limited to a basic few, with the
dying patient's comfort being the principal aim. In view of the
patient's limited life expectancy and vulnerability to pain,
treatment should not be delayed pending laboratory findings.

Continuous pain relief is superior to the sporadic pain
relief provided by inadequate dosage or too long an interval
between doses. The aim of treatment should be to control
pain so that it will not return. This can be compared to the
control of blood sugar in diabetics where the physician does
not wait for symptoms of distress or coma before giving in-
sulin. Breakthrough, or recurring pain is unnecessary pain.
Additionally, recurrence of pain erodes the patient's confidence in his physician while generating anxiety and fear. Constant pain control is achieved through appropriate dosage given
at regular, well-timed intervals.

Ease of administration is a significant consideration because it has substantial impact on the patient's way of life.
The patient taking oral medication is free to move around,
travel in a car and, most importantly, be at home. If pain is
controlled by intravenous injection the patient usually cannot
go home. Injections promote dependence on the person administering the drug. Only 15 percent of patients with terminal cancer receiving hospice care require intramuscular
injections to control their pain at any time.[2] Oral administration eliminates trauma, enables the patient to maintain con-

trol over his own drug administration and helps to retain his options over where to spend his last days.

IMPORTANCE OF PSYCHOLOGICAL FACTORS

Control of pain in a patient suffering from terminal cancer requires comprehensive management which considers all sources of pain whether they be psychological, spiritual, social or physical. Emotional responses have considerable influence on the experience and perception of pain. Dr. Cicely Saunders, Medical Director of St. Christopher's Hospice in England, maintains that a caring figure who listens and tries to understand the patient's sensation of pain is one of the most important factors in the relief of that pain.[3] Kübler-Ross,[4] Hinton[5] and Lamerton[6] agree that the dying have a fundamental need for someone to spend time visiting and listening to them.

Chronic terminal pain can be conceived of as a vicious circle: physical pain arouses anxiety, anxiety generates depression, depression causes insomnia, and insomnia in turn aggravates the physical pain.[7] Control will not be achieved unless pain is viewed with all these components in mind (Fig. 1).

Anxiety and depression are part of the long-term nature of the pain. Patients with terminal cancer whose pain has lasted many months are anxious as they look into the future because they see only an increase in their pain. Anxiety is caused by the meaning of the pain. Acute pains like those of a toothache or childbirth, which physicians learn to manage during medical school, have a purpose in that they indicate a need for action, have a foreseeable end, and frequently hold positive connotations like the birth of a child or the completion of a healing operation. Pain has a sinister meaning for the cancer patient—new or added pain only proclaims physical deterioration.

The degree of perceived pain differs completely between the basically healthy person with acute pain and the cancer patient with severe terminal pain. The patient with advanced cancer perceives pain as occupying total life space. Such pa-

FIGURE 1

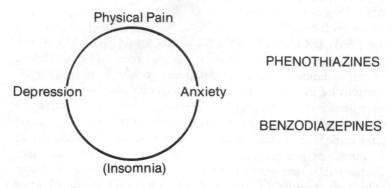

NARCOTICS

Physical Pain

PHENOTHIAZINES

Depression   Anxiety

BENZODIAZEPINES

(Insomnia)

TRICYCLIC
ANTIDEPRESSANTS   NON-BARBITURATE HYPNOTICS

tients often find it difficult to describe the location or the nature of the pain precisely. To questions about the site of pain come responses like "But I'm all pain, Doctor"; "The pain is in my chest and in my back and my arm and my head. Well, it's really all over"; and "I feel as if my body is enclosed in a pressure balloon and the balloon is slowly collapsing, squeezing every bone and every joint in my body as it closes around me." The last statement was made by a woman with a clearly defined site of breast metastasis and source of pain in her lumbar spine. According to her old hospital charts, she had earlier described her pain as a knife sticking into her back. By the time she was admitted to hospice she had developed partial paralysis and a bedsore and had lost all perception of a single pain. Her entire life had become one pain. The physician must take into account the anxiety that these patients are suffering along with the chronic depression caused by chronic pain.

Hinton states that the incidence of anxiety is greater among those who experience a long terminal illness rather than a brief one. He also finds that young people are more anxious during a terminal illness than are older ones, with the greatest anxiety and depression occurring in those dying patients under age 50 with young, dependent children.[8]

Insomnia must be treated resolutely in the patient with pain. Discomfort is often worse at night when the patient is alone with his pain and fear. The cumulative effect of many sleepless, pain-filled nights is a substantial lowering of the pain threshold.

Confidence is the keystone to successful pain management. The patient may initially resist beginning a drug regimen because of a lifelong habit of never giving in or resorting to drugs. Other reasons for resistance may be fear of constipation, addiction, and dreams experienced with certain drugs in the past, or confusion observed in a hospitalized patient. These habits and fears must be identified first of all through sensitive inquiry and an adequate history. Once the block is known it can be dealt with by discussion and education.

Education should include the family so there is an atmosphere of cooperation and support. Hospice nurses spend much of their time with others who help in the home so that the private duty nurse, the visiting nurse and the home health aide understand and support what is being done. Because a visitor may cast doubt on the whole regimen, thereby undermining the positive advantages created by confidence, it is important that the patient and family be able to reach their physician or hospice nurse at any time of the day or night when questions arise. If the questions are not answered speedily and satisfactorily, the patient and family may stop following their physician's advice and abandon the entire carefully constructed regimen.

When dealing with severe pain it is sometimes advantageous to admit the patient to the hospice inpatient facility. Here the patient is affected by much more than drug changes. He is surrounded by a team of people who are completely confident that the pain will be under control before long. Peer support comes from the other patients in the four-bed unit who relate their own individual stories of having pain controlled. The patient sees the others receive their medicine on a regular basis and observes that they are alert and functioning normally.

METHODS OF PAIN CONTROL

General Techniques

Pain control does not begin or end with analgesics; it cannot be achieved merely by writing an order. The therapeutic environment is important: light, flowers, art and, most significantly, caring people. Diversions such as television, radio and talking books or physical and occupational therapy turn attention away from pain and onto other subjects. Pain can be avoided by care in moving a pathologically fractured arm or leg. Heat or ice, pillows and massage all help to ease pain. The patient who described her pain as a pressure balloon was greatly helped by regular two-hourly massage of her paralyzed legs. It is all too easy to concentrate on analgesics and forget that bony pain may respond to radiation. Surgery may be a useful option.

Frequent contact with specialist colleagues and readiness to consult with others will assist the physician in the search for pain control. Control of terminal pain is not usually a matter of exotic new techniques, however, but the correct use of techniques and drugs already known. In mild pain acetomenophin or aspirin is used. For moderate pain codeine or dihydrocodeine will be useful. For severe pain morphine or methadone are the drugs of choice. Table 1 lists the range of pain control methods.[9]

TABLE I

ADDITIONAL ANALGESIC MEASURES

Pharmacological:
  Antibiotics
  Anti-inflammatory drugs
  Glucocorticosteroid

Physical:
  Chemical sprays
  Local heat
  Immobilization
  Jobst compression
  Electrical stimulation

Irradiation

Injections:
  Local anaesthetic
  Peripheral nerve block
  Autonomic nerve block
  Intrathecal block

Neurosurgery:
  Peripheral nerve section
  Cordotomy
  Hypophysectomy

Palliative surgery

Use of Narcotics

Narcotics should be used when non-narcotics, used correctly, fail to control the pain. There should be no hesitation to use morphine or other oral narcotics when other remedies have failed. The severity of the pain must guide the choice of analgesic, not the doctor's estimate of life expectancy, which may be inaccurate. The patient should not be required to wait in pain until the last days or hours of life.

Hospice information is based on studies of the use of oral narcotics for chronic pain in the patient with terminal disease. Generally, most information about narcotic analgesics is related to post-operative patients or those with acute pain as well as studies done on narcotic addicts, animals and parenteral narcotics—all of which may be irrelevant to care for the terminally ill.

Hospice workers have not found narcotic dependence or tolerance to be a problem.[10] Drug dependence can be considered from two aspects: psychological and physical. Psychological dependence is prevented by the use of oral drugs and regular administration. It is of cardinal importance that the patient should not have to ask continually for relief from the threat or presence of pain. Psychological dependence occurs most commonly when a patient is put on p.r.n. ("as necessary") injections in inadequate dosage. Each request becomes a reminder of the dependence on drugs and the person who administers them. Stewart Alsop, in his book *Stay of Execution*,[11] graphically describes this situation in his own terminal illness. If the analgesic is given regularly, the spiral of self-perpetuating pain, dependence and misery is never started.

Physical dependence is not a problem in the patient with limited life expectancy. Physical dependence does not prevent reduction of dose or complete cessation of drug therapy if the disease goes into remission.

Patients do not develop tolerance to narcotics if the dose is precisely adjusted to the degree of pain the patient is experiencing. Patients can remain pain-free on the same dose for many weeks or months. Typical of patients with terminal cancer is a 62-year-old man with lung cancer and subsequent spread of the disease through metastatic lesions who took large daily doses of oral narcotic for 35 weeks. With the exception of the first two days when the pain was being brought under control, the dose fluctuated between 140 and 270 milligrams of oral diamorphine daily. The dose did not increase continuously in staircase fashion and he died without injections: tolerance was not a factor.[12]

The commonly used doses are not always optimal for terminal pain management. Doses which are appropriate for one route of administration are often too high or too low for another due to differences in absorption, distribution and metabolism. Optimal doses of narcotic analgesics for patients with a terminal disease must be determined by titration of the dose to its effect. This is one of the reasons why ordering narcotics in an oral mix is so useful. The physician has a finer control and can titrate the liquid more closely than when using tablets.

Narcotic side effects should receive appropriate management promptly. Sedation can be avoided by finding the gap between continuous pain relief and the onset of drowsiness. This precise dosage, reached by careful titration, can sometimes be a matter of only one or two milligrams, but these few make all the difference. Constipation is so common that a narcotic should never be prescribed without concomitant attention to the bowels. A stool softener, a peristaltic agent which promotes bowel action and, at times, addition of bran to the diet counteract the constipating effect of the narcotics. Nausea and vomiting are prevented by the use of phenothiazines with the narcotic.

Precision Dosage and Timing.
Administration of analgesics in regular and adequate doses provides the continuous preventive relief of skillful pain management. This method uses smaller drug doses, minimizes side effects and allows the dose to be increased as the disease progresses. Occasionally pain returns in less than four hours. This problem can be overcome by (1) increasing the regular dose, (2) decreasing the time interval to three hours or (3) by giving a non-narcotic analgesic between doses. Perhaps a

trusted favorite from an earlier stage in the illness will be useful at this time. The physician can ascertain the correct course of action by asking the patient the following questions:

"Does the medicine ever take the pain away completely?"

"Does the pain return before it is time for the next dose of medicine?"

If the answer to the first question is no, then the dose must be increased. If the answer to the second question is yes, then the time interval should be decreased. If the patient is already approaching the limit of oral dosage, which is 100 milligrams of morphine by mouth every four hours, the correct choice of action would probably be the addition of a non-narcotic analgesic. An analgesic with anti-inflammatory action might be particularly desirable if the problem is bony pain or other pain aggravated by inflammation.

"Four hourly p.r.n." has no place in the treatment of persistent pain. Medication must be given regularly as protection from returning pain. Therefore the physician must know the pharmacology of the drug being used. For example, meperidine or Demerol is effective for an average of two to three hours.[13] The common order given is Demerol every four hours or every six hours. This is insufficient since it condemns the patient to be uncovered by analgesic for at least three hours out of every six. Meperidine and alfaproline are narcotics with short term action. Morphine and heroin (diamorphine) have a four-hour duration. Narcotics with longer action are methadone and levodromeran.

Patients are often given inadequate prescriptions of analgesics. Although 50 milligrams of Demerol by mouth is not a sufficient dose in the average adult it is still in common use.[14] Inadequate dose often results from the interchange of narcotics without proper attention to relative equianalgesic dosage. Again, the result is that the patient is in pain. For example, patients are admitted to the hospital who are taking two or three Percodan every two hours in an unsuccessful attempt to get pain relief. The order is then changed to a small amount of morphine by a house officer who thinks he or she is doing something very dramatic. The change to a small dose of morphine is insufficient, however, since Percodan contains

several analgesic ingredients including the narcotic oxyco-
done, an analogue of codeine. Although codeine and oxyco-
done do not provide as profound an analgesia as morphine, a
patient who has been taking large doses of Percodan will not
find a small dose of morphine to be a satisfactory substitute,
much less an improvement.

Morphine Dosage

An initial dose of morphine may be 10 milligrams every four
hours by mouth. The sedative effect of morphine wears off in
two to three days and can be largely avoided by starting in this
way with a small dose which is increased gradually. The dose
is increased at 48-hour intervals by 5 milligram increments
until control is obtained. If sedation is not a problem, the dose
can be increased more rapidly. Once pain is controlled, the
dose is stabilized and continued every four hours to prevent
recurrence of pain. In the inpatient hospice facility the physician has the advantage of a trained 24-hour team administering the medicines with confidence and making skilled
observations about their effects. In hospice, the physician
writes the narcotic order within a dosage range, for example,
morphine 10 to 20 milligrams every four hours. The nurse
can then vary the dose according to the patient's need at the
time.

Oral narcotics can be given usefully when dissolved in
a syrup base. The "Hospice Mix" is prepared as follows:

> Morphine 5-90 mgs.
> Cherry Syrup to 10 mls.
> Prochlorperazine (Compazine) 5 mgs.

A sample prescription would be:

> Morphine/Cherry Mix 10 mls. every four hours
> Compazine 5 mgs. every four hours

Although this standard mix contains one milligram morphine
sulfate per cc, more concentrated solutions can be prepared
with two, three, four or five milligrams per cc. The strength

of the solution should be clearly labelled.

This Hospice Mix is derived from the classic Brompton's Cocktail used in Britain. The Brompton's Cocktail is a liquid formulation of heroin, cocaine, alcohol, syrup and chloroform water. American hospices have found that the Hospice Mix has similar effectiveness. Some hospice physicians in England, such as Robert Twycross at Sir Michael Sobell House in Oxford, have also eliminated the cocaine and chloroform water.[15] In May, 1977, Dr. Saunders at St. Christopher's Hospice changed to a simple morphine mixture as the narcotic of first choice.[16]

In the rare patient needing high dose injections, heroin is useful because of its high solubility, but it is not necessary for good analgesia in the majority of patients. Twycross has shown that, used orally in equianalgesic doses on a regular regimen with adjuvant, or supportive, drugs, which enhance their action, morphine and heroin are equally suitable agents in terminal cancer.[17]

Adjuvant Drug Use

For patients with insomnia, the hypnotic drug must be chosen with care. Flurazepan or Dalmane is often useful, as is chloral hydrate. Barbiturates should be avoided. They have great potential for drug interactions with many other cerebral depressants. Barbiturates should not be used when the patient is at home. Although the suicide rate in patients facing death is not greater than that for the normal population, the physician must remember that the barbiturates will be available to the bereaved family in the medicine cabinet. Suicide is a definite possibility during the first year of bereavement.[18]

If the patient is receiving adequate nighttime sedation and sufficient analgesic doses during the day, it is often not necessary to wake the patient for the 2:00 a.m. dose. However, a 2:00 a.m. dose may be necessary if the pain is very severe, requiring a high narcotic level throughout the 24 hours. An early morning dose is also indicated if the patient wakes in the morning with pain. It is easier to keep the pain suppressed in this way than to counter it in the morning. When the patient is at home it is advisable to pour the medication the night before and set it at the bedside so the patient can take it himself. This allows the primary care relative to sleep through the night.

Judgment is required in treatment of depression. Depression, as Kübler-Ross has observed, may be an appropriate psychological response as the patient realizes he is dying.[19] Necessary grief work may be performed by the patient during this stage. It is inappropriate to use an antidepressant to treat all depressed patients with a terminal illness. However, a tricyclic antidepressant, such as amitriptyline (Elavil), can be an important part of the pain regimen. The addition of this drug can lift the pain threshold sufficiently to remove the last vestiges of pain.

If a tricyclic antidepressant is used, the physician can take advantage of its short term sedative action by giving all or most of the daily dose at night. It is not necessary to give a tricyclic three times a day although that is a common prescription. In the patient already taking a regular narcotic and phenothiazine, the addition of a daytime antidepressant is frequently too sedative.

Dying patients react to some drugs in the same way as the elderly, particularly to hypnotics and tricyclic antidepressants. Special watch must be kept for sedation and confusion as these may occur at an unexpectedly low dose.

Other anxiolytic drugs such as the benzodiazepines, Valium and Librium, may be used in combination with a phenothiazine or, very rarely, alone with the narcotic. An example of the latter situation would be where no antiemetic effect was required, but cerebral secondaries make the effect of the benzodiazepines useful. Another situation occurs when muscle spasms are a significant contributor to the pain picture.

Phenothiazine Concomitants

When a narcotic is prescribed, a phenothiazine should be ordered with it. Phenothiazines are useful adjuvant drugs for the following reasons:

    1. Phenothiazines potentiate the action of the narcotic, allowing a lower dose of narcotic.

    2. Phenothiazines are antiemetic and counteract the emetic properties of oral narcotics.

    3. Phenothiazines are tranquilizers. Their use addresses the anxiety of pain. [20]

    4. Phenothiazine syrup can be a convenient vehicle in which to dissolve the narcotic.

Care must be taken in the choice of syrup in which to dissolve the narcotic since not all flavors disguise the bitter taste effectively.

The selection of phenothiazine must be made with thorough knowledge of both their different side chain structures and the effect of these side chains on the drug's action.

If more sedation is required, a propylamino derivative may be used. Drugs with this side chain include chlorpromazine (Thorazine) and methotrimeprazine (Lovoprome). The latter drug is purported to possess analgesic activity of its own.[21] It is reserved for inpatient use because it is a sedative that is only available for intramuscular administration and produces orthostatic hypotension, an abnormal fall in blood pressure.

Taking Drugs at Home

Providing the Hospice Mix at home necessitates careful attention to the physical and mental capabilities of the patient and family. Somebody, perhaps a neighbor or relative who lives nearby, must be able to pour an accurate amount of the liquid. Alternatively, a hospice volunteer can come in once every 24 hours and pour out doses. It is helpful to pour individual doses into small brown bottles. Then all the family has to do is unscrew the bottle and give the patient the medicine.

Sometimes the family members are afraid of being responsible for handling a narcotic medicine. In this situation, it is most effective to educate by example. The family becomes accustomed to seeing the hospice staff or volunteer pouring the medicine. They see how simple it is and gradually begin to do it themselves. This is the same role model technique that is so effective in teaching new staff and volunteers their work.

It is essential to make sure that the patient and family know enough about the use of the medicine and accurate ways of measuring. A spoonful means different things to different people. One family member with a slight tremor substituted a soupspoon for a teaspoon to facilitate measuring.

A medication schedule is an extremely helpful tool in the home. Patients with terminal disease are often receiving several drugs concurrently. With so many other things to think about as a result of having somebody sick in the house, the family becomes quickly confused about administration of medications. A card should be used which contains spaces for the names of each drug, the time that each drug dose should be taken, the reason for each drug and any additional comments. This same form can include space for the patient to check off the times at which medication was actually taken. This may seem like extra paperwork, but the hospice staff often find that the patient or relative is proud to present carefully kept records.

Each patient is an individual, each family is unique, and both should be treated as such. The hospice approach to pain control in terminal illness should be seen as variations on a basic theme. Effective pain control is possible using available medical knowledge and with careful attention given to the many factors that comprise pain. No patient should want to die because of the pain he is suffering.

The author wishes to thank Cornelia Chaffin for editorial assistance and Jill Phipps for secretarial help.

NOTES

1. R. G. Twycross, "Relief of Terminal Pain," *British Medical Journal*, 4 (1975), pp. 212-214.
2. S. A. Lack, "Management of Chronic Pain." Unpublished.
3. C. M. Saunders, "The Care of the Terminal Stages of Cancer," *Annals of the Royal College of Surgeons*, Supplement to Vol. 41, 1967.
4. E. Kübler-Ross, *On Death and Dying* (New York: Macmillan Co., 1969).
5. J. Hinton, "Talking with People about to Die," *British Medical Journal*, 3 (1974), pp. 25-27.
6. R. Lamerton, *Care of the Dying* (Priority Press Ltd., 1973).

7. R. Melzack, *The Puzzle of Pain* (Harmondsworth, England: Penguin, 1973), p. 142.
8. J. Hinton, "The Physical and Mental Distress of the Dying," *Quarterly Journal of Medicine*, 32 (1963), p. 1.
9. R. G. Twycross, "Relief of Terminal Pain," *British Medical Journal*, 4 (1975), pp. 212-214.
10. R. G. Twycross, "Clinical Experience with Diamorphine in Advanced Malignant Disease," *International Journal of Clinical Pharmacology, Therapy, and Toxicology*, 9:3 (1974).
11. S. Alsop, *Stay of Execution* (Philadelphia: Lippincott, 1973).
12. R. G. Twycross, "Clinical Experience with Diamorphine in Advanced Malignant Disease," pp. 184-198.
13. L. S. Goodman and A. Gilman, *The Pharmacological Basis of Therapeutics* (New York: Macmillan Co., 1975).
14. R. M. Marks and E. J. Sachar, "Undertreatment of Medical Inpatients with Narcotic Analgesics," *Annals of Internal Medicine*, 78:2 (1973), pp. 173-181.
15. R. G. Twycross, "Choice of Strong Analgesic in Terminal Cancer: Diamorphine or Morphine?" *Pain*, 3 (1977), pp. 93-104.
16. C. Saunders, Personal Communication, May, 1977.
17. R. G. Twycross, "Choice of Strong Analgesic in Terminal Cancer: Diamorphine or Morphine?"
18. S. C. Jacobs and A. Ostfeld, "An Epidemiological Review of the Mortality of Bereavement," *Psychosomatic Medicine*, 39 (1977), pp. 344-357.
19. E. Kübler-Ross, *On Death and Dying*.
20. S. A. Lack, "The Hospice Concept—The Adult with Advanced Cancer," reprinted from Proceedings of the American Cancer Society's Second National Conference on Human Values and Cancer, Chicago, Ill., Sept. 7-9, 1977.

IX
Case History

Palliative Care Service,
Royal Victoria Hospital, Montreal

Reproduced with permission from the 1976 Royal Victoria Hospital Palliative Care Service Report, pp. 213-254.

Royal Victoria Hospital   APPENDIX 12
REQUEST FOR CONSULTATION

TO: PALLIATIVE CARE SERVICE , Home Care
_____Consultant_____ _____Service_____

FROM: _____ 00001
_____Doctor In Charge of Case_____ Licence No.

Mrs. Mary Doe
100 Blank Street
Montreal, P.Q.

PLEASE SEE AND

( ) ACCEPT TRANSFER TO YOUR SERVICE
( ) CONSULT AND FOLLOW WITH ME

( ) SUBMIT WRITTEN CONSUL-
TATION ONLY
( ) CONSULT AND ORDER
INVESTIGATION
( ) CONSULT AND ORDER
THERAPY

REPORT OF
CONSULTATION   DATE Dec. 1st, 1975   TIME 2 P.M.   NO. 28870

C O P Y

F O R

R E C O R D S

Thank you for asking me to see this pleasant woman with cancer
breast and metastases to lungs and bones.

L Radical Mastectomy   June 1974

Adrenalectomy, Oophorectomy Sept 1974

Radiotherapy to Bony Mets Oct - Dec 1974
and since Aug 1975

Chemotherapy Oct 1974 - Oct 1975 - Now Discontinued
(Triple Therapy)

Actinomycin given this week on experimental basis.

This woman worked until 4 weeks ago. She is now confined
to room, getting to bathroom is an effort, dyspnea is
moderate to severe - intermittent chest pain - using Codeine
30 mg prn. Present findings - tachypnea 30-40/min. dry cough
and audible wheeze.

Plan: still wants to be home, will follow regularly -
        - Continue humidifier, nasal O_2
        - Use Codeine 30 mg q4h regularly
        - Home Care Nurse to visit 2x week

_____ M.D.
Consultant's Signature

REASON FOR
CONSULTATION
DATE SENT   TO
CONSULTANT _____ SERVICE P.C.S. NO. 28870

48 yrs. female cancer breast--shortness of breath, increasing pain
Please see re Home Care

DOCTOR
OR
NURSE   ➤   DETACH 3RD PORTION FOR
RECORD PROGRESS NOTES.
IMPORTANT
Requested by _____ M.D.

Form - 707122

PCS - Domiciliary Service

<u>PATIENT ASSESSMENT</u>   Page 1

NAME: <u>Mrs. Mary Doe</u>   DATE: <u>December 2, 1975</u>
ADDRESS: <u>100 Blank Street, Montreal, P.Q.</u>   PHONE: <u>200-1000</u>
PHYSICIAN: <u>Dr. Roe</u>   PHONE: <u>100-2000</u>
DIAGNOSIS: <u>**Cancer breast**</u>
NURSING CLASSIFICATION: <u>2b home</u>
BIRTHDATE: <u>2-2-28</u>   WELFARE #:
DOM. CARE ADMISSION DATE: <u>Dec 2, 1975</u>   OLD AGE SECURITY #:
INSURANCE: LIFE: <u>No</u> HEALTH: <u>Blue Cross</u>
FAMILY CHURCH; NAME: <u>United Church</u>
MINISTER: <u>Rev. Smith</u>   PHONE:
WILL: <u>Yes</u>
FUNERAL ARRANGEMENTS: <u>Not yet</u>

1. FAMILY CONSTELLATION: (Names, Addresses and Telephone Numbers)
   <u>John Doe, husband - office: 111-2222</u>
   <u>Lucy Doe, daughter - 17</u>
   <u>Henry Doe, son - 21</u>

2. OTHER PERSONS:
   <u>Mrs. M. Brown, 101 Blank Street, Montreal, P.Q., 200-1001, neighbor</u>

3. STATUS: <u>2b home</u> ADMIT: <u>**Palliative Care Unit**</u> DR.
   CHANGE OF STATUS:_____DATE:_____ADMIT:_____DR.
   1st DOM. CARE DISCHARGE DATE: <u>Dec. 26</u>   TO:<u>**Palliative Care Unit**</u>
   2nd DOM. CARE ADMISSION DATE:_____STATUS:
   2nd DOM. CARE DISCHARGE DATE:_____TO:
   DATE OF DEATH: <u>Dec. 29, 1975</u>   PLACE OF DEATH: <u>**Palliative Care Unit**</u>

SIGNATURE: Domiciliary RN

CASE HISTORY 93

PCS - Domiciliary Service

PATIENT ASSESSMENT continued   Page 2

NAME: Mary Doe   DATE: Dec. 2, 1975

1. PAST HISTORY:
   Physical Findings: Ca (L) breast, extremely dyspnic, edematous (L) arm, chest
   pain is more severe and relatively constant. She has started to take Demerol,
   takes pm as well as codeine. The pain is worse on (R) ant. chest wall.
   Tabs prn.

2. PHYSICAL:
   Bath, Grooming, Personal Hygiene: Good
   Mobility: **Shortness of breath on slightest exertion**
   Elimination: Ex-Lax regularly
   Communication Sensory: Alert
   Skin: Good
   Sleep: Insomnia at times
3. NUTRITION:
   Therapeutic: None
   Appetite: Fair
   Fluid Balance: Good
4. PAIN CONTROL:
   Region: Chest
   Quality: 1-3
   Occurrence: Intermittent
5. PSYCHOSOCIAL:
   Patient: Tearful at times, aware of disease, worries about children,
   frightened by shortness of breath

6. PSYCHOSOCIAL:
   Family and Others: Husband discusses illness openly with wife, denies prognosis
   to children, who suspect something serious is wrong but are afraid to ask.

7. RESOURCES:

PCS- Domiciliary Service

VISIT REPORT

NAME: Mary Doe   DATE: Dec. 2, 1975

NURSING CLASSIFICATION: 2b   OTHERWISE: HOSPITAL ____ HOME _X_

Visited Mrs. Doe for the first time today- A very pleasant lady, lying in bed propped up by 3 pillows. She spoke very openly of her illness and cried when she talked about leaving her husband and children. Her husband was at work while I was there but her 17 y.o. daughter had stayed home from school with a "sore throat" - Mrs. Doe insisted Lucy leave the room while we talked and told me "I don't want her and Henry to know how bad it is just yet, there's plenty of time to tell them later". Mrs. Doe said neither she nor her husband could discuss her illness with the children, although they could talk about it between themselves - Mrs. Doe said she wasn't frightened of death but she was scared of pain and really panicked when she was shortness of breath.

I arranged to have a portable oxygen set delivered and ordered a hospital bed from the Red Cross. I told Mrs. Doe I would be back in 3 days and would bring along our physiotherapist to show her breathing excercises to help her sh. of br.

After consultation with P.C.S. physician we have discontinued Codeine & Demerol & begun Brompton Mixture with 5 mg of morphine & 5 mg of Stemetil q4h. We also will arrange for a chest X-Ray.

SIGNATURE: Domiciliary RN

PCS- Domiciliary Service

<u>VISIT REPORT</u>

NAME: <u>Mary Doe</u>   DATE: <u>Dec. 5, 1975</u>

NURSING CLASSIFICATION: <u>2B</u>   OTHERWISE: HOSPITAL <u>X</u> HOME ___

<u>Mrs. Doe was sitting in a chair in the living room when we arrived. She says her</u>
<u>sh. o br.</u> has not improved but her pain is less since she started taking the Brompton
<u>5mg</u> Q4h and we began Colace and Senekot to prevent constipation. The physio showed
her some breathing excercises and told her what to do when she has acute **sh. of br.**
attacks. Mr. Doe came home while we were there and was shown how to give his wife
skin care as her back is beginning to show reddened areas. He seems very supportive
and willing to do anything to help his wife. He said he felt better knowing that
there was someone he could call in an emergency.

Volunteer drove her in for chest X-Ray yesterday afternoon. Our physician reviewed
X-Ray with radiologist this AM and apparently there are new destructive lesions on
(R) ant. ribs as well as a small (R) pleural effusion. Radiotherapy was consulted
but felt further radiation was impossible since this area had already received
maximum dose. The oncologist agreed that the pleural effusion was too small for
thoracentesis. Thus our present means of symptomatic control was agreed upon.

SIGNATURE: <u>Domiciliary RN</u>

PCS- Domiciliary Service

VISIT REPORT

NAME: Mary Doe   DATE: Dec. 8, 1975

NURSING CLASSIFICATION: 2b   OTHERWISE: HOSPITAL ____ HOME _X_

Mrs. Doe was alone when I arrived and immediately broke down in tears because she felt "useless and ugly". Her hair has all fallen out because of Chemotherapy (Actinomycin) and she doesn't know how to deal with her baldness. I showed her how to make a turban and will arrange to get her a wig. She also is worried because Lucy is skipping school and is very moody. I suggested that she should talk openly with Lucy about her illness, and tell Henry when he comes home tomorrow from College for the X-Mas vac. She agreed to talk to her husband and then both would tell the children. Mrs. Doe says her shortness of breath has improved a bit with the exercises and she is sleeping better.

Pain was "breaking through" after 3 hours so the dose of Brompton was incr. to 10 mg q4h.

We also will try Ventolin inhalations for sudden attacks of bronchospasm associated with cough. We will also give Linctus Codeine 1 tsp. q4-6h to prevent cough.

Dr. X (Oncology) has decided to discontinue all Chemotherapy since disease is progressing rapidly during therapy. No further active therapy aimed at prolongation of survival is planned.

She has no Nausea/Vomiting but her appetite is dec. She still seems very depressed, although when I left she told me how helpful it had been to her to be able to talk out her worries.

SIGNATURE: Domiciliary RN

PCS- Domiciliary Service
                              VISIT REPORT
NAME: Mary Doe   DATE: Dec. 11, 1975
NURSING CLASSIFICATION: 2B   OTHERWISE: HOSPITAL X   HOME ____

Mrs. Doe in a much better mood. She had a good talk with John and the children
and they were all much relieved to have everything out in the open. Lucy went
to Eatons and got her mother a wig and was able to joke about cutting her own
hair off so she could borrow it. Henry, whom I met for the first time seemed very
quiet and upset since he hadn't seen his mother since Sept. and was shocked at how
thin and ill she was. I found Mrs. Doe weaker, she says it is now almost impossible
for her to get to the BR unaided, so I brought her a bed pan, also a sheepskin
since her back still has reddened areas. She is eating soft foods and liquids, her
appetite is failing but remains well hydrated. As I left, Lucy came out to the
car with me and asked if her mother would die. I said yes."When?" "I don't know
exactly but it's weeks rather than months". She told me how much it meant to her
that her parents had told her the truth, she said she had been feeling left out
and that now that she knew, she could make plans to help in the house and with her
mother's care during the X-Mas vac. instead of going skiing as she had planned.

Pain is well controlled during day but at night (R) chest pain makes sleeping difficult. We will increase Brompton   to 15 mg at the 10PM and 2AM doses and leave
the other doses at 10 mg.

Cough and bronchospasm are improved with Linctus Codeine and Ventolin. She is
using O_2 more often for dyspnoea.

                              SIGNATURE: Domiciliary RN

PCS- Domiciliary Service

<u>VISIT REPORT</u>

NAME: Mary Doe   DATE: Dec. 14, 1975

NURSING CLASSIFICATION: 2B   OTHERWISE: HOSPITAL X   HOME ____

Mrs. Doe c/o increased chest pain and difficulty breathing - her feet and legs are both edematous and she says she has no appetite at all but does drink fluids freely - hasn't had BM for 5 days. I gave her a Fleet enema with good return and increased her Colace to 2 cap BID and Senekot to 1 tab BID.

After consultation with physician, we increased Brompton's to 15 mg q4h around the clock and added Hydrochlorothiazide 50 mg qAM for peripheral edema. She seems a bit weaker but less depressed, says her husband and children are very supportive. She's looking forward to having a good "last" Christmas at home with them and seeing her sister and bro-in-law who are coming from Calgary for the holidays. Hopes to be able to stay out of hospital, would like to die at home.

SIGNATURE: _Domiciliary R.N._

PCS- Domiciliary Service
                              VISIT REPORT

NAME: Mary Doe   DATE: Dec. 17, 1975

NURSING CLASSIFICATION: 2B   OTHERWISE: HOSPITAL _____ HOME X

Mrs. Doe is pain free, her peripheral edema has decreased. However, her cough is
worse and is productive of yellow sputum. Sh. of br. remains moderate to severe--
has not been out of bed for past 2 days. Neighbor, Mrs. Brown was with her. She
seemed very concerned at Mrs. Doe's condition and has been popping in several times
a day to help Lucy with the cooking and house work. Mrs. Doe is worried about
Henry, who stays away from home till 1 or 2 a.m. every day and avoids talking to
the rest of his family. He doesn't stay with his mother for more than a minute or
two and is no help at all in the house.

Mrs. Doe seems to be gradually deteriorating. She eats almost no solids, but still
takes fluids freely.

I will discuss case with Palliative Care Unit physician

                         SIGNATURE: Domiciliary RN

PCS- Domiciliary Service

VISIT REPORT

NAME: Mary Doe   DATE: Dec. 17, 1975

NURSING CLASSIFICATION: 2B   OTHERWISE: HOSPITAL X   HOME ____

14^{00} hrs.

Home visit made this aft. on request of R.N. who found Mrs. Doe's condition deteriorating. Pain well controlled on Brompton 15 mg q4h but now she has severe
sh. of br.even at rest and for last 24 hrs a cough productive of yellow sputum.
Temp. 39° per rectum.

        O/E
        - cachectic, pale - (N) hydration
        - mouth - dry - coated tongue
        - chest - percussion - incr. dullness in (R) base
                - moist râles auscultated over RLL
                - otherwise clear
        - otherwise exam (N)

Imp: RLL Pneumonia

Plan: After discussion with Oncologist, it was confirmed that this patient was
in our category 2B and that symptomatic control was the only appropriate goal.

        - To continue with Brompton Mixture, Linctus codeine, O_2
        - Emergency orders written.

SIGNATURE: P.C.S. Physician

PCS- Domiciliary Service

<u>VISIT REPORT</u>

NAME: Mary Doe   DATE: Dec. 18, 1975

NURSING CLASSIFICATION: 2B   OTHERWISE: HOSPITAL   X   HOME ____

Phone Call: 9p.m. - Mr. Doe called to say **wife has been coughing without stopping**
for last few hours. Advised him to increase Linctus Codeine to 2 tsp. q4h. He
talked a long time about how worried he was about Henry's alienation from rest
of family; the visible deterioration of his wife; how he was going to cope with
all the relatives coming for Christmas and what a sad time it would be for all
of them, knowing Mary is dying. He again said how grateful he was that the Domestic
Care Svce existed and that he could talk to us about all his concerns.

SIGNATURE: _Domiciliary RN_

PCS- Domiciliary Service

<u>VISIT REPORT</u>

NAME:<u> Mary Doe </u>   DATE:<u> Dec. 20, 1975 </u>

NURSING CLASSIFICATION:<u> 2B </u>   OTHERWISE: HOSPITAL <u> X </u> HOME <u>   </u>.

Mrs. Doe incontinent of urine x 4 in last 24 hrs - pain free - edema unchanged, vomited x 2 yesterday, coughing productively, sh. of br.-- patient seems very depressed "I'm going to die soon, aren't I?" "Will I choke to death?" "How long can I stay at home, I'm such a burden to my family".

The patient was catheterized with a No. 16 Foley for 300 cc clear urine. The family was taught how to care for this.

The Stemetil in Brompton Mixture was increased to 10 mg q4h to prevent vomiting.

We had a long discussion about the mode of death and the likelihood of a quiet painless pneumonia developing, impossibility of a clear prognosis but that things were going downhill slowly. The conversation appeared to re-assure her and she agreed that she preferred to remain at home.

SIGNATURE:<u> Domiciliary R.N. </u>

PCS- Domiciliary Service

VISIT REPORT

NAME: Mary Doe   DATE: Dec. 24, 1975

NURSING CLASSIFICATION: 2B   OTHERWISE: HOSPITAL X   HOME ____

    Sister and brother-in-law arrived yesterday from Calgary. They were very upset at seeing Mary but glad that they had come and anxious to keep her home through X-Mas.

Vomiting twice a day, keeping only clear fluids down - coughing increasing, s.o.b. increasing, using nasal O_2 prn, says pain decreased since increased Brompton - is so glad to have sister with her as she feels there are things that she needs to clear up with her.

Henry continues to be a problem, he's never home and is sullen and uncooperative. Lucy feels that he can't accept the fact of his mother's dying and is staying away so he won't have to cope with it. Mr. Doe is not sure that he can manage anymore. Although both he and Mary want her to stay at home, he feels inadequate when she has severe coughing spells. He says Mary also feels that Henry is so disturbed by her illness that he might get into trouble by avoiding home so much. We discussed his problem at length and I told him that if he felt totally unable to cope, Mary could be admitted to the Palliative Care Unit. He said he would keep on trying and I reassured him that he could call me at anytime if a crisis arose.

I taught Mr. Doe and patient's sister how to give Stemetil by IM injection and left supply at home for severe episodes of vomiting.

SIGNATURE: Domiciliary R.N.

PCS- Domiciliary Service

<u>VISIT REPORT</u>

NAME: <u>Mary Doe</u>   DATE: <u>Dec. 26, 1975</u>

NURSING CLASSIFICATION: <u>2B</u>   OTHERWISE: HOSPITAL <u>X</u> HOME ____

<u>Mr. Doe called at 8 a.m. to say that Mary had not slept all night, had vomited</u>
<u>many times and choked during a coughing spell. He said that they had both</u>
<u>decided it would be better for her to be admitted to the **Palliative Care Unit** as</u>
<u>she was frightened of choking to death and he was unable to help her. I went to see</u>
<u>them, found Mary in severe respiratory distress and Mr. Doe very upset. After</u>
<u>discussing the situation, we decided Mary would be more comfortable in the</u>
<u>Palliative Care Unit. Arranged for an ambulance, accompanied Mr. and Mrs. Doe to</u>
<u>Palliative Care Unit--admitted at 11 a.m.</u>

SIGNATURE: <u>Domiciliary R.N.</u>

STANDING MEDICATIONS

ID	PD		
2/12	8/12	BROMPTON MIXTURE _q4h_	
		MORPHINE 5mg	
		STEMETIL 5mg	
5/12		COLACE T BID	
5/12		SENEKOT T BID	
8/12	11/12	BROMPTON c̄ MORPHINE 10mg q4h	
8/12		LINCTUS CODEINE T-TT BID q4h	
11/12		BROMPTON c̄ MORPHINE 15mg q4h	
14/12		HYDROCHLOROTHIAZIDE 50mg qAM	

DOE , MRS. MARY
100 BLANK STREET
MONTREAL , QUÉ

Addressograph   709073 REV.

ID	PD	PRN MEDICATIONS
8/12		Codeine 30mg po q4h
8/12		Demerol 50 mg po q4h
8/12		Ventolin inhalations prn
8/12		Stemetil 10mg IM q4h prn

McGill Home Recording Card

NAME: _Mary Doe_   DATE STARTED: _Dec. 3, 1975_

	Morning	Noon	Dinner	Bedtime
M	1	1	2	3
TU	1	0	3	1
W	0	1	1	2
TH	0	0	0	1
F	0	0	0	0
SA	1	1	1	2
SU	1	1	0	1

PLEASE RECORD

1. Pain Intensity ∅:
   0 - no pain
   1 - mild
   2 - discomforting
   3 - distressing
   4 - horrible
   5 - excruciating

2. No. of Analgesics you have taken.

3. Please make note of any unusual symptoms, pains or activities on back of card.

4. Record hours slept in morning column.

PALLIATIVE CARE UNIT

DOE   HISTORY FORM   FEMALE 48

Past Illnesses: 26/12/75

  - Appendectomy 1950
  - $G_2P_2A_0$ - 2 (N) Childbirths
  - No drug sensitivities
  - No other serious illnesses

History of present illnesses:
  a) Diagnosis: Ca (L) breast

  b) Date initial diagnosis: June 1974

  c) Extent of Disease at Diagnosis: (L) breast, axillary nodes

  d) Course, incl. treatment: (L) radical mastectomy - June 1974
                               Adrenalectomy, Oophrectomy - Sept 1974
                               Chemotherapy - 1974 - Oct 1975
                               (triple therapy + Actinomycin)
                               Radiotherapy to bony mets - Oct 1974, Aug 1975

                               (see consult for details)

  e) Present Extent of Disease:

Systems Review - Present Status: Key 1 major problem   3 absent
                                               2 minor problem   4 don't know

		1	2	3	4	Comments
General:	fatigue	X				
	weight change	X				decreased 30 lbs. last 6 months
	open wound			X		
	discharge			X		
	edema		X			pitting to both knees/improved on diuretic
	fistula			X		
	sleep		X			2-3 hrs. at a time, 2° to s.o.b.
Skin:	Jaundice			X		
	tumor			X		
	decubitus ulcers		X			reddened areas on back

Systems Review - Present Status Cont'd   Key   1 major problem   3 absent
                                                      2 minor problem   4 don't know

		1	2	3	4	Comments
Hematopoietic:	Abnormal bleeding			X		
Respiratory:	cough (prod., nonprod)	X				prod. of yellow sputum
						(difficult to clear)
	dyspnea	X				
	hemoptysis			X		
	wheezing		X			on any exertion
Gastroentestinal:	anorexia	X				fluids only
	nausea	X				
	vomiting	X				2 x 1day
	dysphagia			X		
	bowel dysfunction		X			BM every 5-6 days
	bleeding			X		
Genito-urinary:	voiding difficulty	X				catheterized, incontinent
CNS:	headache			X		
	seizures			X		
	paralysis/paresis			X		
	confusion			X		alert but sleepy
Other:						

Pain: Yes X   No ____   COMMENTS

Severity   Mild ___ Moderate ___ Severe _X_ _____

Frequency   OCC ___   Frequent ___ Constant _X_ _____

Medication   Mild ___ Narcotic ___ Brompton _X_ 15 mg q4h. _____
             analgesic

Control   Excellent ___   Fair/good _X_ Poor ___ _____

Location   Head _____   Type   Pleuritic _X_____

             Chest _____X_____   Dull   _X_____

             Bones _____   Sharp   _____

             Abdomen _____   Pressing _____

             Other _____   Aching   _____

Function

 - bedridden, drinks with assistance _____

 - requires O$_2$ _____

 _____

Family History

A) Medical   Father 69 d. CVA 1967 _____

              Mother 50 d. Ca breast 1956 _____

              Sister 46 alive and well _____

              No familial diseases _____

B) Psycho-social   Aware of dx and prognosis, worried about son. _____

              husband - John _____

              son- Henry, 21 _____

              daughter- Lucy, 17 _____

DOE   FEMALE 48

PHYSICAL EXAMINATION

26/12/75

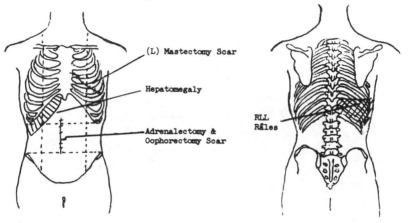

(L) **Mastectomy Scar**

Hepatomegaly

Adrenalectomy &
Oophorectomy Scar

RLL
Râles

- cachectic pale woman of 48 - (N) hydration
- severe respiratory distress at rest
        RR 35/min - using accessory muscles
- denies pain

HEENT - Conj. (N) no icterus
      - Fundi (N) PERL
        Mouth - dry coated tongue
        Neck - NAD

CHEST - RLL râles & dullness to percussion
      - scattered rhonchi throughout both fields
      - well healed (L) mastectomy scar
      - (R) breast palpably (N)

CVS   - S_1S_2 (N) no **murmurs**, no extra sounds
        HR 96/min. reg.

ADB   - slight hepatomegaly, 2cm BCM
      - no other viceromegaly or masses
      - no tenderness

Extremities - + pitting oedema - bilaterally equal

                        (signed) PCS Physician

NURSING HISTORY

FAMILY Mr. John Doe   H-200-1000   Son, Henry
                        Q-111-2222   Daughter, Lucy

WHO TO CONTACT IN EMERGENCY Husband

LANGUAGES SPOKEN English

OCCUPATION Secretary

MENTAL STATUS Alert

PATIENT'S REASON FOR ADMISSION **Shortness of breath, cough, pain control**

DIET HABITS takes fluids only

ELIMINATION HABITS catheter

SKIN CONDITION red areas on back

CONDITION OF TEETH good

HANDICAPS

COMMENTS

NURSING CARE PLAN

PATIENT NEEDS PROBLEMS   NURSING APPROACHES SOLUTIONS

skin care - H_2O mattress

ROOM M464   PATIENT Mrs. Mary Doe   DOCTOR

ROYAL VICTORIA HOSPITAL
MONTREAL, QUEBEC H3A 1A1

DOE

————PROGRESS SHEET————

Dec. 26 1975

PROBLEM LIST

1) Carcinoma of breast

2) Pneumonia RLL

3) Dyspnoea

4) Cough

5) Nausea/Vomiting

6) Pain

7) Bowel Function

8) Urinary Function

9) Decubitus Ulcers

10) Emotional

11) Family

12) Insight

6

DOE

ROYAL VICTORIA HOSPITAL
MONTREAL, QUEBEC H3A 1A1

────**PROGRESS SHEET**────

INITIAL PLANS   (26/12/76)

1) Carcinoma of breast

    - all modalities of therapy attempted

    - 2B-no further active investigations or therapy aimed at prolongation

    or cure planned

2) Pneumonia - RLL

    - dx by clinical exam - not confirmed by X-Ray

    - not causing incr. symptoms

    - after discussion with Oncologist, patient and family, we have elected

    to treat this symptomatically

3) Dyspnoea

    - continue O_2, positioning, re-assurance, humidity

    - may try recliner chair to see if more comfortable

4) Cough

    - continue with Linctus Codeine

    - good mouth care to eliminate tenacious sputum

5) Nausea/Vomiting

    - will continue with Stemetil 10 mg q4h.

    - will also add Cyclizine 50 mg IM BID

6) Pain

    - well controlled on Brompton 15 mg. q4h.

7) Bowel Function

    - continue same dose of Colace & Senekot

    - performed manual disempaction on admission & will receive enema tomorrow

6

ROYAL VICTORIA HOSPITAL
MONTREAL, QUEBEC H3A 1A1

———— **PROGRESS SHEET** ————

8) Urinary Function

       - Foley functioning well

9) Decubitus Ulcer

       - only threatening

       - good skin care for prevention; water mattress, positioning, rubs

10) Emotional

       - see home care notes

11) Family

       - son needs our special attention

12) Insight

       - fully aware of diagnosis & prognosis

ROYAL VICTORIA HOSPITAL
MONTREAL, QUEBEC H3A 1A1

───── **PROGRESS SHEET** ─────

Dec. 26, 1975

Admission: 48 year old woman admitted from home in an ambulance, accompanied by

husband and Dom Care Nurse.

Psychological State: **Patient is aware of diagnosis and prognosis, cried about**

dying and not being able to see her children married. Said she and

her husband have discussed illness openly with children, daughter Lucy

17 is very supportive but son Henry 21, avoids family and is very with-

drawn. Pt. seems accepting of her illness but depressed about son -says

she's frightened of choking to death.
Morphine 15 mg q4h
Current Needs: Brompton Stemetil 10 mg q4h, Hydrochlorothiazide 50 mg qAM,

Linctus Codeine 2 tsp. q4h, Colace 2 BID, Senekot 2 BID, Ventolin inhala-

tions prn, Stemetil 10 mg prn, Dalmane 30 mg qhs.

Diet: Fluids as tolerated, likes ginger-ale.

Family Constellation: Husband John, son Henry 21, daughter Lucy 17, sister and

brother-in-law - Mr. & Mrs. Green.

Religion: United Church, minister Rev. Smith who will visit.

Patient made comfortable on H_2O mattress; back rub given, catheter. draining

well - O_2 mask given, pt. finds it more comfortable. Daughter in to

visit, spoke to Doctor about brother's attitude. Brother called, came

in and spoke with nurse. Cried and said he loved his mother and couldn't

bear to see her so ill. We told him that it would be better for him,

his mother, and the rest of the family if he told his mother how he feels.

He didn't realize how much she worried over his attitude, he said "Why

should they care if I see her or not, I can't make her better."

Eventually, he went in to see Mrs. Doe, he stayed for 2 hours with the

door closed. When he left he thanked us and said that they both felt

ROYAL VICTORIA HOSPITAL
MONTREAL, QUEBEC H3A 1A1

―――― **PROGRESS SHEET** ――――

a lot better

(signed) PCU R.N.

Dec. 27, 1975

7:30-3:30 - Patient had good night, slept till 6 a.m. At 6:30 had episode of severe

sh. of br. coughing N/U and choking. She was very frightened. Nurse

sat with her till she calmed down. Volunteer arranged head-scarf for

her and sat with her x 1 hr. Patient "I'm so glad Henry is O.K. now.

There really isn't much time left for me now is there?". Nurse "No".

"Well, I hope it's soon, I can't take much more of this. I get so

depressed." Long conversation re death and family needs followed.

(signed) PCU R.N.

Dec. 28, 1975

7:30-3:30 - Patient hot--temp. 102.2 sounds very congested--sucking on ice-chips.

Sleeping most of the time responding to name. Family in all day

talking to volunteers in coffee corner. Daughter did a.m. care.

They all take turns sitting by patient's bed holding her hand and

sponging her.

Respiration becoming more labored, suctioned thick mucous, not coughing,

doesn't seem to be in pain, no nausea/vomiting. Visited by minister.

(signed) PCU R.N.

11:00 - Patient's condition stabilized for moment but very little respiratory

reserve. Dyspnoea slightly increased, cough well controlled. No

complaints of pain. O/E R.R. 35/min. regular

H.R. 100/min. regular

6

ROYAL VICTORIA HOSPITAL
MONTREAL, QUEBEC H3A 1A1

──── **PROGRESS SHEET** ────

Colour - pale - (N) hydration

Chest - moist râles in RLL

- scattered rhonchi throughout both fields

Plan: continue same régime.

(signed) PCS Physician

Dec. 29, 1975

7:30-3:30 - Family spent night in Unit. **Patient not responding to stimuli, very**

congested, suctioned x 3. Respirations very shallow and labored-

14:30 - **Patient died peacefully in the presence of her husband and children.**

14:45 - **Patient examined and pronounced dead.**

(signed) PCU R.N.

PCS Physician

6

PCU PATIENT DATA SHEET

Part A - To be filled out on patient's first PCU contact

I. Demographic Data -

Patient name Mary Doe

Telephone No. 200-1000

Address 100 Blank St.

         Montreal, P.Q.

Date of first
PCU contact Dec. 1, 1975

Unit No. 10-10-10

Medicare No. 347921

Medicare No. of key person 219743

Study Number 142

Age 48
      (at 1st contact with PCU)

Sex   M____(1) F X (2)

Race   W X (2) B____(2) Other____(3)

Marital Status

        Single_____(1)
        Married X (2)
        Widowed_____(3)
        D/S_____(4)

Religion Prot.

Importance of religion to patient

        Very____(1)   Somehwat X (2)   Not at all____(3)

Maternal Tongue

        English X (1)   Italian____(3)   Other____(5)
        French____(2)   Greek_____(4)

| 1 | 2 | 3 |
| 4 | 5 |

| 6 |

| 7 |

| 8 |

| 9 |

| 10 |

-2-

Major occupation in life

    Secretary

        Blue collar worker_____(1)
        White collar worker___X_____(2)
        Professional_____(3)
        Student_____(4)
        Housewife_____(5)
        Other_____(6)
        None_____(7)

11

At beginning of present illness, patient was

        Engaged in an occupation___X__(1)
        Retired_____(2)

12

II. Financial Situation

Highest yearly family income_____

        < 5,000_____(1)
        5 - 9,999_____(2)
        10-14,999__X_(3)
        15-19,999____(4)
        20+_____(5)

13

Since patient's illness began, yearly family income has:

        Increased_____(1)
        Remained stable_____(2)
        Decreased up to 25%_____(3)
        Decreased from 26-50%_X_(4)
        Decreased > 50%_____(5)

14

At time of 1st PCU contact patient financially
supports others
             Yes_____(1)   No_X_(2)

15

Patient has life insurance
             Yes_____(1)   No_X_(2)

16

At time of first PCU contact, patient is
concerned about financial situation

17

        Not at all____X____(1)
        Slightly_____(2)
        Quite a bit_____(3)
        A great deal_____(4)

-3-

III. Key Person

Major key person is
Spouse___X___(1)   18
Sibling_____(2)
Offspring_____(3)
Other_____(4)   (State relationship)
                       _____

Occupation of key person at first PCU contact

_____Salesman_____

Retired_____(1)
Housewife_____(2)   19
Blue collar_____(3)
White collar_____X____(4)
Professional_____(5)
Student_____(6)
Other_____(7)
None_____(8)

Has key person altered payable work since patient became ill?

No_____X_____(1)
Yes, began work_____(2)   20
Yes, stopped work_____(3)
Yes, increased work____(4)
Yes, decreased work____(5)

IV. Medical Data
Type of Tumor _Ca Breast_____
                                                     21

Extent of proven disease at first contact with PCU

Local_____(1)   22
Regional_____(2)
Widespread_____X_____(3)

Suspected extent of disease at first contact with PCU

Local_____(1)   23
Regional_____(2)
Widespread_____X_____(3)

-4-

Type of therapy prior to contact with PCU

None_____(0)	S&R_____(5)			24
Surgery_____(1)	S&C_____(6)			
Radiotherapy_____(2)	R&C_____(7)			
Chemotherapy_____(3)	S,R,&C___X___(8)			
Immunotherapy_____(4)	Other combination___(9)			

Source of referral
Oncology Day Clinic___X___(1)   25
Radiotherapy Clinic_____(2)
Surgery_____(3)
Medicine_____(4)
Gynecology_____(5)
Other_____(6)   (Describe_____)

V. **First PCU Admission**

Date of Admission__Dec. 26, 1975_____

Referring physician__Dr. Jones_____

Before hospitalization, lived in_____
                                                                     26
Family home or apartment, alone_____(1)
Family home or apartment, with family or others_X_(2)
Nursing home or chronic care facility_____ ___(3)
Other (describe)_____(4)

Mode of hospitalization in PCU
                                                                     27
Transfer from other hospital bed_____(1)
Admitted directly to PCU____X____(2)

Major percipitating reason for admission

Pain control____X____(1)   Other_____(6)
General support (patient)_____(2)   (Describe_____)   28
KP support_____(3)   Combination of 2 or
Too ill to travel_____(4)   more of above____X__(7)
Intractable vomiting____X____(5)

Functional status on admission to PCU

a) Work
   Has worked or carried out usual daily activity on at
   least some days of past week   Yes___(1) No_X_(2)
                                                                     29
b) Bed Status
   Has been out of bed more than six hours daily
   during past week Yes___(1) No_X_(1)
                                                                     30
c) Feeding
   Feeds self without assistance_____(1)
   Requires assistance with feeding___X___(2)
   Fed partly or completely by tubes or
   IV fluids_____(3)   31

-5-

d) Orientation
    Is oriented to time, place and person the
    majority of daylight hours Yes_X_(1) No___(2)   ‾‾
                                                            32

Work of Key person

    Number of days during week prior to admission KP
    has been able to carry on usual activities __7___   ‾‾
                                                0-7   33

VI. To be completed at discharge of patient after first PCU admission

Care given to patient and/or family during hospitalization

    Nursing   Yes__X_(1) No____(2)
    Psychiatric consultation   Yes____(1) No____(2)   —— 34
    Social work   Yes____(1) No____(2)   —— 35
    Chaplin   Yes__X_(1) No____(2)   —— 36
    VON   Yes____(1) No____(2)   —— 37
    Housekeeper/babysitter   Yes____(1) No____(2)   —— 38
                                                          —— 39

Therapy given to patient during hospitalization

    Pain medication   __X_(1) ____(2) _____   —— 40
    Anti-emetic   __X_(1) ____(2) _____   —— 41
    Anti-depressant   ____(1) ____(2) _____   —— 42
    Sleeping medication   __X_(1) ____(2) _____   —— 43
    Anti-pruritis   ____(1) ____(2) _____   —— 44
    Anti-neoplastic   ____(1) ____(2) _____   —— 45
    Corticosteroids   ____(1) ____(2) _____   —— 46
    RAdiotherapy   ____(1) ____(2) _____   —— 47
    Nerve block   ____(1) ____(2) _____   —— 48
    Other   ____(1) ____(2) _____   —— 49

Disposition of patient at end of first PCU admission

    Death__X____(1)   ‾‾
    Home_____(2)   50
    Other_____(3) (Describe_____)

Part B - To be filled out at time of patient's death

    Date of diagnosis_June 1974___
          (from part I)
    Date of first PCU contact_Dec. 1975_____

    Date of Death_Dec. 29, 1975_____

    Number of home visits by DOM CARE   0   0   8
                                                  ‾‾ ‾‾ ‾‾
                                                  51 52 53

-6-

Place of Death_____
        PCU_____X_____(1)
        Home_____(2)
        Other_____(3) $\overline{54}$

Number of months between diagnosis and first PCU contact

                18 $\overline{55}$ $\overline{56}$

Number of months between first PCU contact and death

                1 $\overline{57}$ $\overline{58}$

Dates of admission to PCU   Number of hospital days
1st admission_Dec. 26,1975_   _____3_____
2nd admission_____   _____
3rd admission_____   _____

                                       TOTAL___3___

Number of admissions to PCU____1____
                                                                $\overline{59}$
Total number of hospital days in PCU___3___
                                               $\overline{60}$ $\overline{61}$ $\overline{62}$
Part C - To be filled out 3 months after patient's death

        Work of KP
             Occupation of KP
                   Same as before patient's illness

                   Yes__X__(1)   No_____(2) $\overline{63}$

                   If no, present occupation_____

        Number of days during previous week that KP has been able to
        carry on usual activities_____7_____
                                          0-7 $\overline{64}$

Part D - To be filled out 1 year after patient's death

        Longevity of KP

             At one year, KP is   Alive_____(1)
                                      Dead_____(2) $\overline{65}$

        Health care utilization of K
             Number of hospitalizations during previous year _____
             Number of M.D. visits during previous year_____ $\overline{66}$
                                                                $\overline{67}$

INFORMATION REQUIRED FOR DECLARATION OF DEATH

Surname of Deceased: Doe

Maiden Surname, If A Woman: White

All Given or Christian Names: Mary Jane

Street Address: 100 Blank St.

Official Name of Municipality or Township: Montreal

Municipal County: Province: Quebec

Postal Code: H1C 3X6

Date of Birth: Month 2   Day 2   Year 28 . Age 48   Sex F

Birthplace (Province, or Country Outside Canada): Montreal

Citizenship: Canada   Ethnic Origin: English

Number of School Years Completed (Passed): 11

Language Spoken At Home (One Only): English

Marital Status: Single_____ Married X   Year of Marriage_____

        Widowed_____ Year Widowed_____ Divorced_____

        Year Divorced_____ Legally Separated_____ Year_____

        (If Separation Is Not By Court Order, Show As Married)

Full Name of Husband   (Including Maiden Surname of Wife):_____

        John Henry Doe

Year of Birth of Husband   1926

Surname And Given Name of Father: Fred White

Birthplace of Father (Province, or Country Outside Canada): England

Maiden Surname and Given Name of Mother: Alice Black

Birthplace of Mother (Province, or Country Outside Canada): Quebec

Trade, Profession or Kind of Work of Deceased: Secretary

Kind of Industry or Business: Insurance Office

Date Deceased Last Worked At This Occupation: Nov. 1975

Total Years Spent In This Occupation: 7

Disposition of Body: Burial X Cremation_____ Transport outside Quebec_____

Name And Address of Funeral Director:_____

Information Obtained From: John Doe   Relationship to Deceased: husband

        By: P.C.U.   Position: R.N.

BEREAVEMENT COPING ASSESSMENT

KP NAME	John Doe
ADDRESS	100 Blank St.
	Montreal, Que.
PHONES	H. 200-1000 O. 111-2222
MEDICARE NO.	219743
RELATIONSHIP TO PATIENT	husband

DOES KP ACCEPT FOLLOWUP. Yes X   No ___

STAFF MEMBER MOST
CLOSELY INVOLVED _____

OTHERS NEEDING FOLLOWUP/HELP: None
(show names, addresses, relationships)

DATE OF DEATH: Dec. 29, 1975

Lucy Doe 17, daughter
Henry Doe 21, son - will need more help than rest of family

COMMENTS: (include details of help already being given)

QUESTIONNAIRE SUMMARY

A.	4
B.	2
C.	1
D.	2
E.	1
F.	2
G.	1
H.	1
TOTAL	14

QUESTIONNAIRE   (circle one item in each section)

A. Age of KP
= (only if KP is spouse)
1. 75 +
2. 66-75
3. 56-65
④ 46-55
5. 15-45

B. Occupation of principal wage earner of KP's family
1. Profes. & Exec.
② Semi-Profes.
3. Office & Cler.
4. Skilled Manual
5. Semi-skilled "
6. Unskilled   "

C. Length of KP's preparation for patient's death
① Fully prepared for long time
2. Fully prepared for less than 2 weeks
3. Partially prepared
4. Totally unprepared

D. Clinging or Pining
1. Never
② Seldom
3. Moderate
4. Frequent
5. Constant
6. Constant & Intense

E. Anger
① None (or Normal)
2. Mild irritation
3. Moderate, occasional outbursts
4. Severe, spoiling relationships
5. Extreme - always bitter

F. Self Reproach
1. None
② Mild, vague & general
3. Moderate - some self reproach
4. Severe - preoccupation, self blame
5. Extreme - major problem

G. Family
① Warm, will give full support
2. Doubtful
3. Supportive but live at distance
4. Not supportive
5. No family

H. How will KP cope?
① Well. Normal grief and recovery without special help.
2. Fair. Probably manage without special help.
3. Doubtful. May need special help.
4. Badly. Requires special help.
5. Very Badly. Requires urgent help.

BEREAVEMENT FOLLOW-UP CHECKLIST

NAME: John Doe, Lucy, Henry

DATE: Jan 27, 1976

DATE OF BEREAVEMENT: Dec. 29, 1975

I. Vital function

    (1) appetite   better ( )   worse ( )   unchanged (X)

    (2) sleep   better ( )   worse ( )   unchanged (X)

    (3) weight   increased (lbs)   decreased (lbs)

                                                       unchanged (X)

II. Supportive contact

    (1) Initiated by: staff (X)   Key Person ( )

    (2) Time spent: 1 1/2 hrs.

    (3) Extent of social contacts: fair

    (4) Quality of social contacts: good

    (5) Contact with Clergy: slight

    (6) Contact with family: good

III. Current status regarding:

    (1) housing   better ( )   worse ( )   unchanged (X)

    (2) occupation   better ( )   worse ( )   unchanged (x)

    (3) finances   better ( )   worse ( )   unchanged (x)

IV. Psychological status:

    (1) Mood - depressed off and on

        If depression mentioned - ask:

        "Have you been so discouraged that you considered suicide?"

                Yes ( )   No (X)

    (2) Feelings of guilt: Yes ( )   No (X)

    (3) "When you lose someone you care for deeply, it may afterwards

        seem that they are not really gone, or that they have returned

        in some way.

        Have you experienced anything like this since your loss?

        (a) Hallucination ("vision")   (b) dream

                auditory - hears her moving around in bedroom when he's
                               in living room
                visual -

                        (c) delusions (actual belief)

      When I called Mr. Doe, he was eager to have me come and see him.
I went to the house at 8p.m., he and both children were there. I stayed
till 9:30. Mr. D. said the funeral had been very well attended. Many
friends and neighbors came and his wife's family stayed on for 10 days
after the funeral. He feels that he and the children have become much
closer since Mary's death and they all have been able to share their
feelings openly. Henry goes back to school tomorrow and Mr. Doe feels
that he has come to terms with his mother's death and although he's sad,
he does go out with his friends and brings them back to the house as well.
Lucy cried as she talked about her mother's illness, she feels the burden
of running the house-hold, even though they now have a house keeper who
comes in 3 times a week. Lucy said she still expects to see her mother
when she comes in from school and has to remind herself each time that
"Mom's gone for good now." They all spoke at length about how helpful
they felt the P.C.S. had been to them and how glad they were that Mary had
been at home for her last Christmas. "That's what she wanted and we couldn't
have done it without your help."

      Mr. Doe said that he's been feeling better since he went back to work,
but that with Henry away at school and Lucy out with friends, he'll feel
lonely in the evenings. However, he plans to go back to his bowling league
and also go away at Easter with the children. He said the worst experience
he had was when Mary's sister cleaned out her clothes 10 days after she died.
"It made it seem so final, somehow."

V. Interview

    Report:

         I feel that they are all coping well with their grief and
    beginning to make adjustments and re-enter daily life. The three
    of them seemed very close and loving and supportive and I feel that
    no further visits are necessary, although I said I would call in a
    couple of months to see how they were. As I left, each one kissed
    me and thanked me for taking the trouble to think of them and see
    them.
                              (signed) PCS Bereavement Nurse

PART III

THE ELEMENTS OF ORGANIZATION

X

Three Approaches to Patient Care: Hospice, Nursing Homes, and Hospitals

SARAH BURGER, R.N.

The chart on page 132 outlines the differences between hospice, hospital, and nursing home care. It is a quick reference and is the basis for the more detailed description of the three types of care discussed in this chapter. The differences far outweigh the similarities. Each of the three types of institutions provides care for a specific set of problems with specific outcomes. Although 80 percent of the care of the terminally ill in this country occurs in hospitals and nursing homes, it is the thesis of this chapter that hospice care is far more appropriate for both humanitarian and financial reasons.

"The time for terminal care is reached when all active treatment of the patient's disease becomes ineffective and irrelevant to his needs."[1] Terminal care usually takes place during the last three to six months before death. A comparison of the care given in nursing homes, hospitals, and hospices will demonstrate why a hospice program can better meet the needs of the terminally ill.

A hospital is designed to treat acute illnesses using highly technical and aggressive means. It is designed to prolong life. A patient is admitted with a particular set of symptoms to be diagnosed and treated. The hoped-for outcome is discharge to the community with the original problem under control. For-

Sarah Burger is presently Vice-President of the Washington Hospice Society, Inc., an organization which she helped to found. She is also coauthor of a book entitled Living in a Nursing Home: A Complete Guide for Residents, Relatives and Friends.

CHART I

	HOSPITAL	NURSING HOME	HOSPICE-INPATIENT
PROBLEM	Acute illness	Chronic illness	Terminal illness
OUTCOME	Discharge to community or institution—97.5%; death—2.5%	Discharge to community or lower level of care—74.2%; or death—25.8%	Death; bereavement
CARE GIVEN	Institutional: hospital	Institutional: nursing home	Home care with institutional backup
CARE GIVEN BY	Hierarchy of: Physician Registered Nurse Licensed Practical Nurse Nursing Assistant Auxiliary personnel	Circle of: Physician Registered Nurse Licensed Practical Nurse Nursing Assistant Auxiliary personnel	Team of: Physicians Nurses Social Workers Volunteers Clergy
FAMILY INVOLVEMENT	Peripheral	Some involvement	Great involvement of family incorporated in giving care
LENGTH OF STAY	7.3 days (1977)	84 days	Projected 10-12 days
ENVIRONMENT OF INSTITUTION	Sterile	Somewhat homelike but distinctly institutional	Homey; non-institutional
COST OF STAY	$173.98/day (1977); about 50% of cost is for personnel	$24.04/day (1977); about 55% of the cost is for personnel	Approximately $100/day (1977); more than 60% of the cost is for personnel
SOURCE OF DATA	(Health Care Financing Administration, Division of Hospital Services, United States Department of Health, Education and Welfare)	(National Center for Health Statistics, United States Department of Health, Education and Welfare)	(Hospice, Inc., New Haven, Connecticut)

tunately, the system is technologically efficient so that tests and treatments are carried out quickly and the patient discharged in a short time, the average hospital stay being 7.3 days.

But what happens to the patient who cannot be cured? Can this efficient diagnostic treatment system meet the special needs of the dying patient? Should hospitals have to treat a group of patients who do not fit the purpose for which the system was established? The experience of Dr. Elisabeth Kübler-Ross in 1965 is illustrative of the place of the dying in the hospital setting. When she asked to interview a dying patient in a large Chicago hospital, she was struck by the response of the physicians and nurses: "The reactions were varied, from stunned looks of disbelief to rather abrupt changes of topic of conversation. . . . It suddenly seemed that there were no dying patients in this huge hospital."[2] Although Dr. Kübler-Ross and others have revolutionized the ways of responding to the needs of the dying patient, little has been done to change the ability of the acute-care hospital to meet the needs of the terminally ill. In hospitals, 97.5 percent of the patients are discharged, while only 2.5 percent die there.

The primary purpose of nursing homes is to rehabilitate patients so that they can return to their community or to a lower level of care. In 1976, 74.2 percent of all nursing home patients were discharged alive, and only 25.8 percent of the patients were either not discharged or died.[3]

Rehabilitative care is also called long-term care, which has been defined as:

> . . . a series of services provided to chronically ill and disabled persons over an extended period of time. Chronic conditions are often gradual in onset and of lifetime duration. Unlike acute illnesses, which occur suddenly and are usually resolved in a relatively short period of time, chronic illnesses are difficult to treat medically except to maintain the status quo or *effect some functional improvement*.[4]

The mean length of stay in nursing homes is 84 days.

The terms "nursing home" and "long-term care institution" suggest that the care given may be more appropriate than hospital care for the terminally ill. Indeed nursing homes are homes which provide nursing care; however, they are mostly "skilled" and "intermediate care" nursing institutions, definitions used by federal and state governments to describe the amount and kind of care given.

A skilled nursing facility (SNF) has a registered nurse in charge seven days a week, twenty-four hours a day. Such nursing homes have a sophisticated paramedical staff geared to rehabilitating patients to their maximum level of independence. The intermediate care facility (ICF) has less sick and more independent patients requiring less intensive professional nursing care. In fact, a registered nurse or a licensed vocational nurse need be on duty only during the day shift, seven days a week. To some extent these institutions can meet the special needs of the dying patient, but because of a rigidity in style of operation (partly due to government regulations) and staffing patterns, a nursing home is often not suitable for a dying patient or his family.

Hospice care, on the other hand, is geared solely to meeting the needs of the dying patient and the family: the dying patient should be free of physical, mental, social, and spiritual pain in order that he may live as fully as possible, hopefully at home with his family.

Statistics show that 76 percent of terminal patients in the United States elect to die at home if appropriate support systems are available.[5] The hospice program is primarily oriented toward home care, and the majority of its patients die at home. If specialized hospice home care was available, three kinds of terminal patients would choose it: 1) patients whose families need a temporary respite from the demands of giving primary care at home; 2) patients who need special treatment for specific symptoms, either physical or mental; and 3) patients who have lived alone or have no suitable person to provide care for them. The hospice offers a home-like environment with few restrictions where appropriate treatment and support is given to the patient and the family in order that he may live as fully as possible in the time remaining.

A hospice does not have either the equipment or staff for diagnosis or curative treatment. In fact, resuscitative equipment simply does not exist in the hospice environment. Should a patient die, he is allowed to do so without last minute attempts at revival. We have mentioned that one basic need of the dying patient is for emotional or psychological support. This support requires extensive time commitments from the staff on an unscheduled basis, and nursing homes do not have sufficient trained people to provide such care.

How do existing federal and state regulations affect the quality of care for the terminally ill and their families? Hospice care is presently unregulated by the federal government, so control is left to the states. The usual state or local dietary, sanitation, and fire safety laws can and must be observed. Nevertheless, the special staffing patterns of hospices, the presence of pets, and unrestricted visiting hours, are all possible under existing state regulations. However, a serious problem concerns financial reimbursement by third party insurers. The states currently may designate a hospice only as a nursing home, a hospital, or an extended care facility. Since the operation of a hospice is significantly different from all three of these institutions, the reimbursement received would not adequately reflect the unique kind of service a hospice provides. Yet without appropriate reimbursement from third parties such as Medicare and Medicaid, a national hospice program cannot be forthcoming.

The difficulty of providing federal regulations was recognized by the former Secretary of Health, Education, and Welfare, Joseph Califano. If regulations are drafted too quickly, without taking into account the operational experience of the existing model hospices, the danger is that appropriate care standards and an accurate basis for reimbursement might not be established. Thus, in his address to the National Hospice Organization's first annual meeting in October, 1978, Secretary Califano said: "Our challenge is to nourish this movement, not force-feed it."

Federal and state regulations for patient safety and cost-effectiveness are complicated and allow institutions very little flexibility. In addition to the necessary high standards of sanitation, there is a system of patient review including utilization review and PSRO (Professional Standards Review Organization). Utilization review is carried out by a committee within the institution; PSRO is carried out on a regional basis. These reviews were established by the federal government to ensure that patients are in hospitals for appropriate reasons. A dying patient not receiving active treatment may be in constant fear of being moved or having his insurance payments cut off because he is in the hospital for inappropriate reasons. Sometimes a patient is kept in the hospital because there is no place to which he can be discharged. How unsettling it must be for the dying individual to be in an institution which not only fails to meet his needs, but which is also trying to place him elsewhere. If insurance payments to hospitals are stopped, the family and patient will suffer financially.

A similar situation exists in nursing homes. The division of nursing homes into ICF's and SNF's refers to both the kind of services given and to the level of payment made by either Medicaid or Medicare (58 percent of nursing home care is paid by these programs). The Utilization Review Committee must decide whether the patient is receiving the appropriate level of care. If he is not, then he will either be moved to an institution that gives appropriate care, or redesignated within the present institution, if it provides both ICF and SNF care. Again, this assessment process contributes to a feeling of uneasiness when security is important. Thus, in reality, the patient receives care based on federal/state-mandated reimbursement rates rather than on the care needed. In addition no payment is made for bereavement care for the family in either hospitals or nursing homes. Bereavement care is crucial to the hospice program and may be fairly intensive during the first year after the death of a family member.

Who actually takes care of the terminally ill patient and his family in the three types of institutions? The following diagrams show, in a simplified way, differences in staff patterns and authority.

It is safe to say that in all three situations the patient is of primary importance. But there the similarity ends. The differences exist not only in the decision making, but also in

CHART II

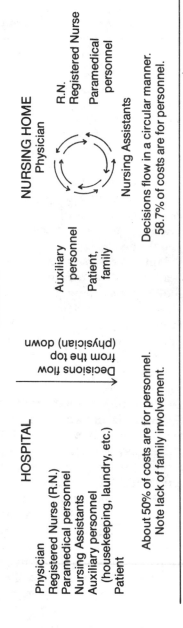

HOSPITAL

Physician
Registered Nurse (R.N.)
Paramedical personnel
Nursing Assistants
Auxiliary personnel
(housekeeping, laundry, etc.)
Patient

Decisions flow from the top (physician) down →

About 50% of costs are for personnel.
Note lack of family involvement.

NURSING HOME

Physician

R.N.
Registered Nurse

Paramedical
personnel

Nursing Assistants

Auxiliary
personnel

Patient,
family

Decisions flow in a circular manner.
58.7% of costs are for personnel.

HOSPICE

Physician, Registered Nurse, Paramedical Personnel, Volunteer, Patient, Family

Decisions are made by a team with the patient and family as equal partners.

Approximately 60% of costs are expected to be for personnel.

quantity and quality of the members of each of the professions involved in care.

Hospital care is directed by the physicians, for it is they who have the training and expertise to properly diagnose and treat. A physician writes orders, often on a daily basis, and expects them to be carried out by the rest of the hospital personnel. The registered nurse oversees each patient unit, making sure the orders are completed efficiently. The doctor and nurse consult one another frequently about the patient. Actual daily personal care may be given by primary care nurses (R.N.'s), Licensed Practical Nurses (L.P.N.'s), or nursing assistants under the supervision of an R.N.

Paramedical personnel have frequent short contacts with patients in hospitals. A patient undergoing diagnostic tests may visit two or three different departments in a single day. One often hears hospital patients joke about needing to go home for a rest after a hospital stay! Who hasn't visited a friend or relative in the hospital only to discover the bed empty? Upon finding a nurse, one learns that the person is at X-ray and won't return for some indeterminate length of time. But in order to arrive at a diagnosis and appropriate treatment as quickly as possible, hospitals must follow schedules. Clearly, there is little opportunity for consulting the patient about how he would like his stay in the hospital to be arranged. For the patient in need of diagnosis and treatment, the American hospital is an efficient (if impersonal) system.

The terminal patient, however, does not generally need efficient diagnostic services. Diagnosis and treatment are pertinent only insofar as they apply to palliative care. J. M. Hinton's study of patients dying in a busy general hospital shows how difficult it is for staff to meet the emotional needs of the dying patient.[6] (See also chapter three, "Ten Bad Days Among the Dying.") Physicians are trained to cure; death is not "curable." Until recently, medical and nursing education has not included courses on dying and death. Curriculum changes are now being made so that students learn something about terminal care and the ramifications for patient, family, and staff. Until recently, however, most faculty were not qualified by education or experience to teach about terminal illness.

The patient who is dying is often lonely and frightened and needs people who are willing to sit, listen, and talk with him. Hospital volunteers could perform such tasks, but presently they are only given jobs of transportation, delivering messages or flowers, or supervising the bookmobile. Clergy and social workers can sometimes give this kind of comfort to patients, particularly if they are employed by the hospital. However, there is no hospital training for volunteers, clergy, and indeed for most medical professionals to carry on this work. Nor is training given for personnel to help the family before, during, and after the patient's death.

The personnel in nursing homes may provide a more caring and relaxed atmosphere for the dying patient and his family. The attending physician does not make day-to-day decisions about patient care as he does in the hospital. The R.N. is primarily responsible for assuring that the total needs of the patient and family are met, though 80 percent of the actual personal care is given by untrained, unlicensed nursing assistants. There is much excellent care, but only because the majority of nursing assistants try very hard. Nursing assistants are not trained to care for terminally ill patients or their families. Backed by force of federal regulation, Medicare- and Medicaid-certified homes are required to provide in-service training to nursing assistants. However, a nursing assistant may work for an extended period of time with no training other than a brief orientation. There is no control at present over the quality of the in-service training and only three states (Minnesota, Iowa, and Oregon) require a specific training curriculum. Only fourteen states require tests for nursing assistants before or soon after employment. Progress toward required training and possible certification of the nursing assistants is being made by the industry; however, years will pass before these important people receive the level of expertise their work requires. Who knows when "caring for the terminally ill" might be included in an in-service course? Yet about 25 percent of the patients in a typical nursing home will die there.

Nursing homes are using volunteers more and more. A few homes offer training so that volunteers will be more confident in their roles. Although few participate in actual patient care, volunteers provide services such as social contact, running errands, reading aloud, and even sometimes playing an advocacy role for the patient vis-à-vis the doctors and nursing home staff. The amount of time clergy give to calling in nursing homes varies, but unlike hospitals, nursing homes frequently have worship services which are open to all residents.

Although nursing home routine is not as strict as hospital routine, each day has a structure. The times for meals, baths, treatments, and activities depend on employee availability, and most of the staff is on duty during the day shift. The main meal may be served at 11:30 a.m. or 4:30 p.m. For many people, to change from a 6:30 p.m. dinner to a 4:30 p.m. dinner is very upsetting. These may seem like minor problems to those of us who still control our lives, but to patients confined to an institution, they become matters of enormous importance. Dr. Robert Kastenbaum describes the effects of institutionalization:

> Because institutional living is not the typical living arrangement for people in our society, the impact on the individual who enters an institution or other congregate facility can be traumatic in the extreme.[7]

Kastenbaum makes three further points about the effects of institutionalization: the absence of friends or significant people and familiar objects can be devastating, producing a feeling of defeat and uselessness; the security of well-learned patterns of daily living and of familiar surroundings are swept away; and

> ... the newly institutionalized person becomes anchorless, often rejected and unloved; rudderless, without family or familiar guidelines. In a milieu quite foreign to his experiences, he frequently adapts by bizarre defensive behavior that further isolates him from his fellows.[8]

The isolation can then extend to his own family.

Nursing homes are becoming more and more aware of

the importance of the family in the rehabilitative process. Thus, one sees more of a "circle of care" in the nursing home, as opposed to the hierarchical situation seen in the hospital. Still, one must keep in mind that care is given by unlicensed, untrained personnel who may not be prepared to meet the complicated needs of the terminally ill patient and family, except by doing what comes from the heart. In a discussion of patient care with some nursing assistants recently, the importance of the role of the family was brought up. They were quick to point out that they were not allowed to talk with the families! Although this situation does not exist in all nursing homes, it is a typical administrative restriction. The assistants described their reaction as follows: "We feel as if our hands are cut off."

In order to live life to the fullest, a person must retain as much *control* over his or her life as possible. Hospice care is specifically tailored to make this control a reality for the patient. All decisions are made by a team working together as equals with the patient exercising final authority. Each member of the team brings his or her own expertise. The physician must be an expert on pain control and relief of symptoms, and must be a good diagnostician in order to distinguish between symptoms caused by terminal illness and any which develop unrelated to that illness. The nurse, whether an R.N. or L.P.N., must be attuned to the same things as the physician. His or her care of patient and family must be unhurried and unstructured, given on a one-to-one basis. If there is a need to be met, it must be met immediately, not later or tomorrow. Terminal illness causes much stress and, in order for patient and family to keep their equilibrium, they deserve immediate attention.

The role of clergy and volunteers is unique in hospice care. They too are equal partners with the patient, his family, the physician, the social worker, and others in planning and providing care. Sometimes the volunteer, who is rigorously screened and trained, becomes the most important person to the patient and/or family. To put this in perspective, hospice volunteers are presently better prepared to help the terminally ill than are nursing assistants in nursing homes. Volunteers are trained prior to service rather than on the job, and they also receive in-service training.

Another significant characteristic of hospice care is that family members are as intimately involved as they desire. Bereavement studies show that families who help with the care of their relatives have a less complicated bereavement period. Thus, in the hospice, the family is welcome day or night. They may actually give physical care to the patient—feed, bathe, walk—or whatever they feel comfortable doing. Provision is often made for privacy so that private and/or sexual needs of families can be maintained as desired. This is not true in a hospital, where only certain family members can visit during fixed hours. Is it realistic to deny dying patients visits from children or grandchildren simply because the children are under twelve? Should visits to such a patient be restricted to two hours in the afternoon and two hours in the evening? There are health and safety reasons for restricting visitors in a hospital, but the dying patient needs family and friends whenever he or she has the strength.

Nursing homes, once again, fall somewhere in between the rigidity of the hospital and the flexibility of the hospice. Nursing homes usually permit visiting for a six to eight hour period during the day or evening. However, if a nursing home is truly a "home," with nursing care, there should be no restrictions. Children are usually allowed to visit, although sometimes families feel it is "too scary" for them to see so many old, sick people. Privacy or conjugal visiting is an issue which has been regulated by the federal government. In the patient bill of rights it states:

> . . . the patient, if married, is assured privacy for visits from his/her spouse; if both are inpatients in a facility, they are permitted to share a room, unless medically contraindicated (as documented by the attending physician on the medical record).[9]

This ruling depends on the goodwill of the administration and staff of each nursing home, for it is very difficult for federal or state inspectors to enforce. Compliance is irregular and often not controlled by the patient.

Many administrators of nursing homes are realizing that the family is an important adjunct to success in the planning of care. Still, little is done to make the family a partner in care. Two things work against such activity. First, the family may think they should not help because they are paying for that care. Second, nursing homes are in a beleaguered state; witness the Senate Subcommittee on Long-Term Care Reports of 1976, entitled "Nursing Home Care in the United States: Failure in Public Policy." The supporting papers have such titles as "Drugs in Nursing Homes: Misuse, High Costs and Kickbacks"; "Doctors in Nursing Homes: The Shunned Responsibilities"; and "Nurses in Nursing Homes: The Heavy Burden (The Reliance on Untrained and Unlicensed Personnel)." Care has improved since these reports were issued, but there is more to be done. Administrators continue to be guarded and defensive on many issues affecting patient care.

The physical environment differs between hospitals, nursing homes, and hospices. The very fact of an institution produces some barriers between those outside and those inside. Hospices in England and in the United States have tried to break down these barriers and minimize the patient's physical removal from his home and family. Hospice, Inc. of New Haven was built as a hospice and therefore the design of the building itself was carefully planned around the specific comfort and needs of the dying and their families. Not all hospices are or will be built to such specifications. In many instances, hospices will be located in an existing building or a wing of a hospital. In all cases, however, there is an attempt to relieve the dreariness of institutionalization by judicious use of color, light, windows, and furnishings. Life is to be lived in a hospice and everything possible is done to reach that goal. The environment is not sterile as in a hospital. Patients are encouraged to bring important possessions with them. While many nursing homes attempt this, regulations do not permit them the flexibility of a hospice.

This chapter has described the many differences in the care of the terminally ill in three kinds of institutions—hospitals, nursing homes, and hospices. It has been shown that a hospital is usually inappropriate, the nursing home is inappropriate as now operated, and that the hospice is designed specifically for care of the dying patient and his family. Cost is the final issue. Of the three, hospitals are most expensive, nursing homes least expensive, and hospice lies somewhere in between (see Chart 1). The reason for these differences is that hospitals have very high overhead costs with sophisticated, expensive diagnostic and treatment equipment costs which have to be shared in the cost per patient per day. Hospices, on the other hand, have large personnel costs. Nursing homes have neither the high equipment costs nor the professional personnel costs. They rely on minimum wage, nonprofessional personnel as described above.

The three kinds of institutions—hospital, nursing home, and hospice—provide very different kinds of care to patients with specific types of needs. The hospital provides cure or control of acute diseases; the nursing home provides rehabilitative and preventive care for chronic diseases; and hospice provides care for the terminally ill. There is a clear and cogent need for each of the three institutions in our society.

NOTES

1. Cicely Saunders and Charles A. Garfield, editors, *Psychosocial Care of the Dying Patient* (McGraw-Hill, Inc., New York, 1978), p. 22.
2. Elisabeth Kübler-Ross, *On Death and Dying* (Macmillan Publishing Company, Inc., New York, 1969), p. 23.
3. *Advance Data,* Vital and Health Statistics of the National Center for Health Statistics, United States Department of Health, Education and Welfare, Public Health Service, #35, Sept. 6, 1978, p. 5.
4. *Long-Term Care for the Elderly and Disabled,* the Congress of the United States, Congressional Budget Office, Washington, D.C., February 1977, p. 1.
5. John W. Abbott, "Hospice," *Aging* (Nov.-Dec. 1978, No. 289-290), p. 40.
6. J. M. Hinton, *Dying* (Penguin Books, Harmondsworth, England), chapter 8.
7. Robert Kastenbaum, *New Thoughts on Old Age* (Springer Publishing Company, Inc., New York, 1964), p. 207.
8. *Ibid.,* pp. 207, 208.
9. American Health Care Association, *HEW Interpretive Guidelines and Survey Procedures,* Washington, D.C., 1975, p. 11.

XI

A Hospice Program Within an Acute Care Medical Center or Hospital*

NORMAN T. WALTER, M.D., P.H.D.

Hospice care can fit into the mainstream of good hospital medical care. To assure that a hospice program can do just that, we developed the following program to satisfy the needs of the patients, their families, and their physicians. We have a separate unit within our hospital or medical center *and* a home care program to assist the family in maintaining a patient at home when that is possible. We have knit together a team of nurses, aides, volunteers, and social workers who can work under the direction of the patients' own physicians to provide both excellent medical care and psychosocial support for the period of the terminal illness as well as the period of bereavement.

GOAL

Our goal was to create a program for the care of patients and their families who are facing a terminal illness. Our program had to:

Dr. Walter is a Senior Partner of the Permanente Medical Group in Hayward, California, Attending Surgeon at the Kaiser Foundation Hospital, and Project Director and Medical Director of the Kaiser-Permanente Hayward Hospice Pilot Project.

*This presentation is taken in part from a report to the Board of Directors of the Kaiser Foundation Hospitals and to The Permanente Medical Group, the organizations which generously provided funds and staff to support the Kaiser-Permanente Hayward Hospice Pilot Project.

145

1. Address itself to patient/family needs.

2. Fit within the mainstream of good medical care.

3. Support, rather than disrupt, the continuity of care and the doctor-patient relationship.

4. Avoid unnecessary replication of facilities and equipment.

5. Make maximum use of existing medical and community services.

6. Be integrated with all other necessary programs of the medical center and have an identity and integrity comparable to other integrated services departments (e.g., CCU, ICU, Intensive Care Nursery, etc.).

7. Be satisfactory to patients, families, physicians, nurses, and medical center personnel.

8. Be cost-effective.

RATIONALE

If we could successfully accomplish the above, then the program could be rapidly replicated in many similar medical centers, thus upgrading the quality of care for a large number of people.

Another benefit would be that we would have demonstrated that hospice programs can be conceived and implemented within Acute Care Medical Centers, thus giving medical services planners an option which many believed did not exist. What we will have established is that hospice programs need not necessarily have separate, detached, facilities in order to survive.

SPECIFIC AREAS OF CONCERN CALLING FOR SPECIFIC STRATEGIES

The development of a five-point educational program for our physicians:

1. To upgrade symptom management and control skills.

2. To recognize when it is appropriate to turn to palliative care strategies rather than strategies for cure, and also to recognize when a patient is probably within three to six months of death.

3. To recognize how a hospice program can help the physician better understand and cope with the patient and family needs and to utilize community resources in their support.

4. To help physicians discuss the reality of impending death with patients and their families in ways which are helpful.

5. To help physicians learn to be one of the leaders in an expanded team which includes social workers, volunteers, ministers, nurses, the family, and others. Each profession makes a unique and necessary contribution to the welfare of the patient.

Educational program for nurses, social workers, and volunteers:

1. To demonstrate that hospice work is practical, that it really benefits both patients and the staff.

2. To learn first and foremost to do for the patient and family what needs to be done—whether it be to break up a fecal impaction, provide for food or feeding, or teach patients and families how to look after themselves and care for each other.

3. To accept that "counseling" *per se* has a small place in the care of the terminally ill and to recognize that death is not a psychiatric illness. Skills need to be sharpened in the area of "listening, observing, and communicating."

4. To learn to earn the "friendship and trust" of the patient and family. Earning the patient's trust is a major factor in the prevention of the sense of isolation that has been so often reported as one of the most distressing events of traditional terminal care.

5. To learn how to work as an integrated team of attending physicians, nurses, aides, volunteers, social

workers, psychotherapists, home care nurses, and so forth. Developing a team takes time and effort, but it has very handsome payoffs in terms of the range of skills and continuity which can be provided for patients and families.

6. To remove the "mystique" surrounding the care of the terminally ill. We need to reaffirm that the care of the terminally ill is neither awesome nor fearful. We need to reaffirm that providing such care can be peaceful and soul-satisfying.

Medical Center Administration and Nursing
Administration Issues

If we had opted to create one major hospice referral center, it would of necessity have become geographically remote from many of our patients and their families, as well as from physicians. In order to keep the family deeply involved in the caring program, it is necessary to keep the support systems within reasonable proximity (20-25 miles or 30-45 minutes).

If we had opted to develop a single referral center, it would become necessary to develop a group of medical specialists for the care of the terminally ill. Upgrading the understanding and the skills of all physicians and nurses in the needs and care of the terminally ill would better serve both physicians and patients. This is a far better choice than that of developing another "specialty" which would tend to further fragment care to patients and create even greater discontinuity of service with all of its attendant hazards and discomfitures.

Medical center administrators must not allow their traditional priorities to stand in the way of the hospice program. In other words, the traditional techniques of cost containment by virtue of minimal nurse/patient staffing ratios and high bed utilization figures must be reassessed. The use of such techniques mitigates chances of success of a hospice program.

First, administrators had to be convinced that the quality of care for terminally ill patients and their families could be improved. The entire administrative hierarchy needed to understand the philosophy and priorities of the hospice program. It was important that they were not just "desirous" or "interested" in supporting the hospice program, but *committed* to the concepts and the philosophy of the program and therefore willing to make *sacrifices* to see the program succeed. It was necessary to get the administrative team committed to support the program for a finite period of time (two years), and then to agree to an evaluation of the program.

The medical center administration agreed to a number of things:

1. Not to consider an empty bed an anathema.

2. To allow us to *organize* and *integrate* "services and place" utilization in a somewhat different fashion than had been done traditionally.

3. To allow us to engage in trial staffing patterns to determine what works best.

4. To allow us to designate an area of the hospital which would be redecorated and refurnished in a home-like way for patients and families.

5. To allow us to remove all visiting restrictions.

6. To provide a bed for relatives wanting to spend the night with the patient.

7. To make it possible for families to eat together if desired.

The nursing office agreed to allow for the training of a "core group" of nurses and aides interested in working with the terminally ill. The inpatient unit would then be staffed with people from this "core-group." The training and orientation to hospice, its goals and objectives, was presented to all members of the medical center—administrative, supervisory, and service personnel, including engineers, housekeepers, dietitians, pharmacists, and gardeners.

We also developed a Hospice Home Care Team which provides for services in the home as well as visits to patients who may be living in an extended-care facility.

Hospice patients are given first priority for the use of inpatient beds in the hospice unit area of the hospital. At times, when most of our hospice program patients are at home and bed space is short elsewhere in the hospital, we have used hospice beds for "Med-Surg" patients. Conversely, when there was greater hospice inpatient need than the unit could support, patients were accommodated in "Med-Surg" beds. This maximized our integration within the medical center. This also served to keep our nursing staff skilled in traditional kinds of care.

We have developed staffing strategies which allow us to have our second or third trained member of the nursing team able to work elsewhere in the hospital if the hospice inpatient unit has few patients. This serves to spread the skills, philosophy, and humanity underlying the program to other parts of the medical center. As a result we have seen significant positive impact in areas like the Intensive Care Nursery, Emergency Room, Intensive Care Unit, and Coronary Care Unit, where crises tend to occur precipitously and hospice-trained nurses have been able to demonstrate excellent support for family and other involved staff.

One of our hopes in having a hospice program in a hospital is that the basic humanism of the program would radiate to other parts of the hospital, mitigating the often-heard complaints of impersonal use of technology and lack of individual caring—familiar complaints in busy hospitals.

The "acuity of care" need is established on a shift-by-shift basis and the inpatient unit is staffed accordingly. The senior nursing person in the unit is a highly skilled, hospice-oriented registered nurse (R.N.). We have found that our inpatients are among those most often requiring highly skilled nursing services. If the inpatient population is four or above, a second hospice-oriented person is assigned. It may be an R.N., an aide, or a Licensed Vocational Nurse, depending upon the judgment of the Medical-Hospice nursing supervisor. She may at times of need call for a third person to be assigned to the unit, based upon a "needs-assessment." The judgment of the supervisor is predicated upon patient and family needs as she perceives them during her rounds.

The administration has allowed time for regular informal nurse get-togethers to discuss patient care problems, team problems, and program problems. This has been so successful that other units at the hospital are beginning to consider using this strategy.

Medical Center Issues: Who—When—How to Admit to the Program

The patient's attending physician must make a judgment that the patient is afflicted with an illness which is expected to end life within approximately six months, and that maintaining or improving the quality of life for that patient is to be a major goal for the intervening period. The patients and families who are accepted into the program need to accept the concept that palliative care is the major goal of future medical interventions.

The various parties involved must understand and accept the "no code blue" philosophy: that there will be no heroic or desperate attempts at resuscitation or prolonging life. The patient and/or family must be able to grasp the inappropriateness of a "code blue" philosophy in the future care of the patient. However, each individual patient's situation and philosophy determines the appropriate strategy. In many instances such recognition serves as a benchmark of patient-family understanding.

In order to admit a patient to the program, the attending physician will have to determine that the patient fulfills the above criteria, and will then call any one of six designated physicians who must make a similar judgment on the merits of the diagnosis. The consulting physician then notifies the program secretary or admitting office to admit the patient into the program—either to the inpatient unit or for home care. The patient's attending physician writes the transfer orders as well as the further care orders if the patient is elsewhere in the hospital and is to be moved to the hospice unit, or the home care orders for the home care nurse. *The patient's attending physician continues to write all subsequent orders on the patient and controls the patient's medical management.* The hospice physicians serve primarily as consultants for developing strategies for symptom control and management.

WHAT DOES THE PROGRAM PROVIDE?

Inpatient Unit

The inpatient unit serves two functions. It provides:

1. Patient beds for achieving symptom control when this cannot be accomplished on an outpatient or at-home basis.
2. Family respite for brief periods if needed.

Home Care Program

The home care program serves three functions. It provides:

1. Support to the family in caring for the patient in the home.
2. Continuity in physician's care.
3. Skilled home care nursing supervision.

The home care team serves to keep the patient's physician, as well as the remainder of the hospice team, informed of the patient and the family's current status, problems, and potential resolutions.

Medical Center Education

The hospice program has provided a series of programs for all parts of the hospital to heighten awareness of the needs of the terminally-ill patients and their families. The goals and objectives of the program have been disseminated throughout the hospital, throughout the clinic area, and into all supporting service areas.

Patient/Family Weekly Status Review

There is a regular, formal, weekly review of all patients and family members being cared for in the hospice program, both inpatient and outpatient. This review constitutes a situation report, strategy planning conference, and bereavement follow-up report. Present at this weekly review are:

1. Hospice program coordinator.
2. Nurse responsible for providing the home care service.

3. Key nurse on the day shift on the inpatient unit.
4. Medical-Hospice nursing supervisor.
5. Social worker.
6. Home health aide.
7. Physician in charge of the Home Care Program (an internist).
8. Medical director of the hospice program (surgeon).
9. Guest participants—other nurses, aides, volunteers, physicians, clergy.

Hospice Staff and Support Strategies
First and foremost in the development of the hospice program is the selection process. The hospice coordinator, along with the supervisor of nurses and director of volunteers, interviews all potential nurses, aides, and volunteers as a pre-staffing screening device. A great deal of screening out is done at this level.

There is preparatory indoctrination of all potential staff members and volunteers. This includes a presentation of history, hospice philosophy, the need for a hospice program, our particular program structure, our expectations, and our strategies for coping with stress. It must be emphasized that in our screening and in our indoctrination programs we do try to indicate that the kinds of people we are looking for are people who have skills, compassion, and an ability to accept a variety of different patient attitudes toward death.

We provide for continuing in-service education on a regular basis.

For hospice program staff and volunteers, we have social get-togethers to aid communication and understanding. For hospice program family and friends who are survivors (bereaved), along with available staff, we have provided a number of social get-togethers, especially around holiday time.

It is important to plan for informal meetings to enhance community feeling between staff members and the program coordinator and between the medical director and other members of the staff and volunteers. This leads to a tremendous amount of openness and direct communication between various members of the team. Crisis situations are dealt with directly, not put on a back burner for future meeting agenda items.

Hospice Program Coordinator

The program coordinator should be a person with superb "people" skills and patience, experienced in leadership techniques which are gentle but persuasive; supportive but not stifling; consistent but not rigid. The coordinator needs to be a person who is reliable, dependable, dedicated, and *available*. The coordinator should be a person who does not need to "take over" or "usurp" the duties and responsibilities of others. He or she needs to be able to understand and tolerate conflicts while gently working to avoid them.

The program coordinator provides for the day-to-day management of the program and coordinates and orchestrates the patient's services. The coordinator also serves as liaison between the hospice program and the other medical center departments which are not directly represented on the hospice planning committee or the hospice administrative committee, that is, housekeeping, engineering, dietary, and physiotherapy.

Hospice Medical Director

The medical director must understand the medical community which uses the medical center, and the administrative structure responsible for administrating the medical center. It is also very helpful if this person is respected by both of these communities. The director serves as liaison with the medical staff as well as consultant resource for symptom management strategy.

Hospice Program Administrative Committee

This top-level committee includes the hospice medical director, the hospice program coordinator, the medical and hospice supervisor of nurses, the director of nurses, and the assistant hospital administrator. They meet on a weekly or biweekly basis to discuss the total program, current problems, and who is responsible for resolving them. The committee insures that the program is *integrated* into the medical center activities and lives up to its commitment to patients, family, and staff.

Volunteer Coordinator

The volunteer group is comprised of a dedicated group of individuals who are viewed by the patients and families as their peers. The volunteers gather information through personal contact which can give the other members of the hospice team clearer insight into patient and family needs. Volunteers also provide the rest of the team with support and reassurance which can enhance the morale of the staff. A hospice program cannot reach its full level of achievement without volunteers. They provide patient and family with support in ways and at times when professional teams would be inappropriate and inadequate. The hospice staff views volunteers as peers and as an integral part of the team.

Social Service Department

The social service department provides the program with social workers to work with patients and families. Social services are used as a part of the planning strategy for responding to patient and family needs, arranging for discharge and readmission as needed, as well as being part of the psychosocial support system.

Religious Ministry

Ministerial support is provided on a voluntary basis. Patients of all denominations and of all faiths are encouraged to invite their particular priests or ministers to participate in patients' care as desired.

Physiotherapy, Pharmacology, Dietary, and Support Services

All medical center functions and services are available to the hospice patients as appropriate. Programs for educating the staff of these various departments as to the specific needs of the terminally ill and their families have been carried out and cooperation from these various departments has been outstanding.

SUMMARY AND CONCLUSIONS

The program has now been operating for a year. We have served 125 patients and their families. The problems we have faced have primarily centered around education to improve skills and strategies, and the usual problems of team building and communication. It would appear that these problems are being overcome because acceptance and support of the program by patients, families, physicians, and nursing staff, as well as the entire medical center staff, has been phenomenal.

Since the program stabilized we have not seen any significant or unusual amounts of staff or volunteer disaffection or distress, sometimes referred to as "burn out." This may be due to our careful screening and selection process, our ability to "float" staff out of the program for a while if they desire, our avoidance of the creation of false expectations on the part of the staff, our "support strategies," our ability to be flexible, and our openness in preparing staff for their need to be able to confront uncertainty and to live with it.

At this point there are no real obstacles to the development and success of a hospice program within an acute care medical center as long as the administration, physicians, nurses, and patients share the same goals.

XII

The Connecticut Hospice Volunteer Program

MARJORIE SUE COX

Volunteer services are an essential part of the hospice program in Connecticut. Volunteers established hospice and they continue to be invaluable as direct caregivers, professional consultants, assistants in administration, members of the Board of Directors, and advocates in the community. Through the creativity and commitment of volunteers, other hospices have been established across the United States. This description of the Connecticut volunteer program has been written for the benefit of the newer groups. The model is based on five years of experience in home care, with anticipated inpatient services in October, 1979. It has been designed to change continually as new volunteer services are needed by patients, families, and hospice development.

The Connecticut Hospice has had an organized volunteer program headed by a staff Director of Volunteer Services since April, 1974. During the first year, forty-six volunteers were selected and trained for work with patients and families or for administrative and clerical responsibilities in the hospice offices. As the Hospice Home Care Program developed and expanded its services of caring for patients and families, and of providing information and education programs for the community, the numbers of volunteers and hours of volunteer

Marjorie Sue Cox is Director of Volunteer Services at The Connecticut Hospice, Inc. in New Haven.

service increased. Statistics from annual reports reflect the development of the volunteer program: in 1975, forty-six volunteers recorded 2,223 hours of service; in 1976, sixty-six volunteers recorded 6,086 hours of service; in 1977, seventy-four volunteers recorded 9,849 hours of service; and in 1978, 121 volunteers recorded 12,068 hours of service in all hospice departments.

Volunteers have served in the following categories: (1) receptionists who greet visitors, sort mail, and answer the telephone; (2) public speakers who present the program to community organizations; (3) clerical assistants assigned to departments for tasks such as editing, typing, filing, collating, xeroxing, or data collection; (4) workers who update mailing lists and prepare mass mailings; (5) photographers and writers for special tasks in public information and education; (6) registrars for meetings, conferences, and workshops; (7) hosts and hostesses for special events; (8) library and resource center workers; (9) researchers in community service resources; (10) drivers for errands and volunteer transport; (11) sitters for children of staff and volunteers; (12) leaders who coordinate the volunteer teams assigned to a specific job description; and (13) advisory committee members for planning and evaluation of various aspects of the program.

Volunteers have worked directly with patients and families in the following positions: (1) regularly scheduled visitors assigned to a patient or family member as part of the care team; (2) drivers for escorting and transporting patients and family members to necessary appointments and social outings; (3) drivers for errands such as medicine and supplies, food shopping, laundry, and equipment delivery; (4) assistants for homemaking and home maintenance tasks when fatigue, stress, or finances are causing practical and routine problems; (5) sitters to be with patients or children to allow the primary care person a rest or social break; (6) staff escorts when the provision of care requires two people; (7) professional nurses to supplement staff nurses in the care of patients and families; (8) mental health professionals to supplement and support clinical staff in the counseling and education of families; (9) people with training in pastoral care to supplement and support staff in the planning of an expanded program of pastoral care; (10) physicians to supplement and support staff physicians in the provision of care for patients and families; (11) people with expertise in music, art, handicrafts, and recreation to provide service or consultation when needed; (12) people to communicate in foreign languages and with the deaf to provide service when needed; and (13) bereavement team members to follow families through bereavement with visits and support as needed.

PLANNING HISTORY

Hospice was first organized in 1970 with the selection of a Board of Directors and the appointment of task forces to plan various aspects of the program. Officially incorporated in 1971, hospice relied from its very beginning on volunteers. Professionals from the medical, nursing, social service, and religious disciplines worked with lay community leaders to establish hospice. They volunteered their time and expertise by serving on planning committees, speaking to community groups, and seeking funds for the organization. The sustained commitment of these founders proved that volunteers are reliable if their expertise is needed and used.

In April of 1974, a Director of Volunteer Services was hired as part of the original health care team which included a physician, five nurses, a social worker, and a secretary. The Director of Volunteer Services was selected for a variety of reasons. She had led the initial organization of innovative volunteer programs. She had a background as supervisor of volunteers with expertise gained in coordinating volunteers of varied ages, personalities, and educational levels to maximize their contributions. Having worked in a health care institution, she had gained experience in selection, training, and supervision of volunteers both in their work with health care professionals and in meeting the needs of seriously ill patients and their families.

The Director immediately interviewed volunteer applicants in order to select a core group to participate in the development of the volunteer program. This group of ten men and women included a wide variety of educational levels and backgrounds to represent the various types of skills which would be needed. The staff and volunteers decided that the best way to learn how to give assistance during illness, dying, and grieving would be to ask people who were ill, dying, and grieving what they needed. By listening to patients and families, the paid and unpaid staff helped the patients and their families to identify the problems with which they needed help. The hospice program was designed, in effect, by the consumer.

The core group of volunteers worked closely with the Director and other staff to determine which patient and family needs could be appropriately assigned to volunteers. They also clarified how the volunteer can provide effective service in the total hospice program apart from direct patient/family assistance. Before defining the hospice categories of volunteer service, volunteers surveyed the quality of service provided by other health care and social service agencies which utilize trained volunteers in this community. They learned that this information should be frequently updated as the quality of service varies when personnel change, budgets tighten, or agencies change their priorities. This information enabled hospice to identify categories of service which were needed, to make knowledgeable referrals when appropriate, and to be prepared to fill the gaps in the health services system.

The decision to employ the Director of Volunteer Services as part of the original staff has proven valuable in a program geared to meet the needs of client, staff, and volunteer. By being present from the beginning, volunteers could participate in decisions on the details of procedure and policy development while rendering thousands of hours of patient and family service. Volunteers were also able to participate in interdisciplinary team growth. Attendance at staff in-service education sessions and clinical conferences equipped the core group for helping with the integration of new volunteers. This enrichment of the curriculum for volunteer orientation and training continues in the fifth year of the program.

In August, 1974, the Director of Volunteer Services visited St. Christopher's Hospice and St. Luke's Nursing Home in England to meet with volunteers and their supervisors for observation and consultation. It was evident that patients, families, and paid staff relied on quality volunteer service in roles which were uncommon in English general hospitals. The skills of volunteers were being utilized to enable them to work with the staff sharing both caring tasks and caring relationships. For example, a staff nurse and a trained volunteer would bathe a patient and change the bed together. This allowed the extra time for both to engage in leisure conversation, and to attend to the grooming and comfort details which were important to the patient. The hospices had developed an environment where trust relationships grow between professionals and non-professionals; where patients, family members, volunteers, and staff join together to give and receive care; and where the inevitable blurring of roles reduces interdisciplinary tensions. Hospice personnel feel that this type of teamwork is necessary for the effective care of terminal patients.

To implement the hospice philosophy of care in this country, an organized structure for management of the volunteer program was needed. The utilization of services by lay and professional volunteers required written procedures to define training, reporting, supervision, and responsibility. An administrative manual was written and is kept updated. The manual is a valuable tool for the Director and other administrative staff, particularly for evaluation. The careful development of the volunteer program has provided a solid foundation for services which meet every discipline's standards, helps to keep the cost of health care down, prevents duplication of services, and enhances the total package of care hospice provides.

MANAGEMENT

The Director of Volunteer Services is responsible for the management of the volunteer department. The volunteer department is organized to provide volunteer personnel to supplement staff responsibilities. The Director encourages and cooperates with other staff and volunteers to: (1) ensure that volunteers are utilized as an integral component of the hospice program; (2) set goals and objectives for volunteer services; (3) plan policies and procedures; (4) identify job descriptions for volunteers; (5) select and assign volunteers with consideration for the skills, knowledge, and motivation of the individual and the goals of hospice; (6) provide for the orientation of new volunteers; (7) promote job satisfaction by providing guidance during the early stage of their work and ongoing inservice education; (8) structure the organization to include the supervision and support of volunteer personnel; (9) provide for individual job performance evaluation, growth, and mobility; and (10) structure the organization to provide for volunteer participation in planning and evaluation of the program.

POLICIES

To clarify the purpose and goals of using volunteer services the following policy statements serve as guidelines for implementation of the program:

1. Volunteer services are an integral component of the hospice program. Volunteers supplement and support the paid staff's responsibilities in the provision of care to patients and families by providing services in all hospice departments.

2. Volunteers do not replace paid positions; the patient caseload and administrative goals are determined by the available time and expertise of paid personnel. Volunteers provide additional services which enhance the care of families and augment the work of paid staff in all departments.

3. Quality service is a higher priority than large rosters of volunteers or quantity of hours. The number of new volunteers joining hospice must increase at a rate which enables the maintenance of high levels of communication and continuity of service in all hospice departments.

4. All applicants for volunteer service are interviewed by the Director of Volunteer Services. The only exceptions are special task forces organized by the Board of Directors for specific projects or in situations when the Director of Volunteer Services designates another person to interview for a specific job description.

5. All applicants participate in an orientation course planned by the Director of Volunteer Services or by other personnel designated by the Director. Each course plan is individually designed after assessing the applicant's education, experience, and skills in relation to the mutually agreed upon assignment.

6. Volunteers are assigned to departments by the Director of Volunteer Services with the agreement of the department head. Specialized training and supervision is the responsibility of the department in which the volunteer serves. Volunteers are invited to participate in education opportunities planned for their department and to become involved in the planning, development, and evaluation of department programming.

The rationale for these policies is to insure that volunteers understand the total hospice program before beginning service in one department, and that people are placed in jobs which best utilize their skills and individuality. This encourages commitment, job satisfaction, and a sense of effective integration into the hospice community. Additionally, these policies provide guidelines for a structure which will insure that volunteer service is consistent with hospice goals and with standards set for paid personnel.

RECRUITMENT

The Connecticut Hospice has had a waiting list of volunteer applicants throughout the five years of the organized program. This pool of human resources has been available because of an organizational commitment to public education. The Hospice Department of Public Information coordinates a year-round program of speaking, teaching, and media presentations. Most volunteers have applied for service after hearing or reading about hospice through this educational effort. Many presentations are made to professional groups and as a result hospice attracts health professionals as well as non-professionals. The waiting list does not supply all of the volunteers needed by hospice. For example, because of the success of the national hospice movement, there has always been a need for additional skilled clerical help.

Active recruitment becomes necessary when an unusual skill or talent is required to meet a specific patient or family need or when unpredicted attrition occurs in a particular category of service. Our experience indicates that personal referral from experienced personnel and knowledgeable supporters is an excellent recruitment source. When a specific skill is needed, members of the Hospice Board of Directors, the staff, and the volunteers support the program by recruiting through their other interest groups and contacts in the community.

Another valuable resource for special recruitment is the cooperation between directors of volunteer services in the greater New Haven area. Directors meet to become familiar with each program in order to encourage effective cross referrals. This region is also fortunate in having several organized systems which provide counseling and knowledgeable referral for applicants interested in matching their expertise and time to volunteer service opportunities.

The Friends of Hospice, a statewide auxiliary organized to support hospice, is also a recruitment resource for special task projects. Volunteers are attracted from a broad geographical area because consultation services are available to families throughout Connecticut, and the inpatient hospice facility opening in October 1979, will provide an inpatient care alternative for patients throughout Connecticut.

APPLICATION PROCEDURE

Applicants are initially requested by phone or mail to provide some information about their skills, interests, and experience to enable volunteer department personnel to determine if hospice has an available position which might be appropriate for them. Printed information on the hospice program is mailed to applicants, and they are encouraged to attend an informational presentation on the program before an interview is scheduled. These presentations are scheduled on a regular basis by the Department of Public Information.

The Director of Volunteer Services, or another person

designated by her, is scheduled to meet with each applicant for a two-hour interview. The objectives of the interview are to: 1) provide further information on the hospice program, the philosophy of care, and the organizational structure; 2) discuss service opportunities; 3) discuss the background, interests, and skills of the applicant; 4) learn the reasons why the applicant wishes to volunteer at hospice; 5) complete the application form; and 6) provide the applicant with printed information on hospice and the volunteer program.

The goals of the interview are to give and receive adequate information for a mutual decision on the appropriate placement of the applicant. The Director's primary interest during the interview is in the answers to the following questions: 1) Who is this person? 2) What is the reason for applying? 3) Has the person suffered a major loss, such as the death of a loved one or a divorce? Has the loss been resolved? 4) What would be the ideal volunteer position for the applicant's needs, skills, goals, and motivation? An applicant is encouraged to talk through ideas on the purposes for volunteering, and to participate in a decision on placement. At times, applicants are referred to other institutions or agencies which provide volunteer service opportunities that are more suitable for the individual's available time, skills, and goals.

When applicants with special skills for working in administration, planning, fund-raising, public information, reception, or education express an interest in suggested job descriptions, the Director notifies the appropriate department. An interview is then scheduled with department personnel to discuss the department's goals and organization, details of the job description, and the procedures for training. All new trainees are assigned to a volunteer group leader or directly to a staff person for training supervision.

ORIENTATION COURSE

The orientation course is designed primarily for interviewed applicants who wish to work directly with patients and families, and are likely to be suitable in the opinion of the Director of Volunteer Services. Six to eight applicants meet with the

Director for three sessions to learn more about hospice care and how they might fit into the team, to explore their feelings about disease and death, and to discuss listening techniques. The course is a further opportunity for the applicant and the Director to evaluate the suitability of the individual for direct caregiving before the actual training procedure of travelling into patients' homes with staff. The course protects patients and families from exposure to persons who lack understanding of their problems, protects the caregiving staff from the expense of time and energy on unsuitable applicants, and protects the volunteer from exposure to disease, dying, and grieving without preparation.

During the three small group sessions, the following material is covered:

1. *Hospice Organization.* A brief review of the development of hospice: its philosophy, goals, characteristics, categories of service, criteria for admission, interdisciplinary staff and volunteer expertise, interagency cooperation, organizational structure, volunteer roles, and policies and procedures.

2. *Reading List.* Applicants are required to read *On Death and Dying,* Elisabeth Kübler-Ross; *Questions and Answers on Death and Dying,* Kübler-Ross; *Death—The Final Stage of Growth,* Kübler-Ross; and *Bereavement—Studies of Grief in Adult Life,* Colin Murray Parkes. Volunteers are encouraged to continue reading in the area of their interest, selecting books and articles from the hospice resource center. Reading is discussed during the orientation course.

3. *Feelings.* For a session in exploring personal feelings about death many tools are available, such as planning one's own funeral service or the service for a significant other person. Some individuals have benefited from writing out a newspaper death notice for themselves and sharing their life's accomplishment and next of kin details with the group. One successful method is to assign the following questions for individual thought and group sharing: a) If you could choose when you would die, when would it be? When would you not want to die? Why? b) If you could choose how you would die, how would it be? How would you not choose to die? Why? c)

Thinking of that person with whom you are most close, who would you want to die first? Why? d) What do you fear most about dying? Open discussion of these questions identifies the problem list of the entire patient/family caseload. Using the list, the Director points out the need for the expertise of the entire interdisciplinary team to help patients and families cope with the realities of terminal illness: pain and other symptoms—vomiting, nausea, constipation caused by disease or its treatment, body or mind deterioration, immobility, dependency, loss of self-esteem, loss of control, guilt, unfinished business, unfulfilled dreams, indignity, isolation, and nonproductivity. The patient and family problems are physical, psychological, spiritual, social, and financial.

4. *The Gift of Self.* Hospice has learned that caregivers must keep in touch with their feelings so that they are free to be present to the needs of patients and families. One thought and discussion stimulant which has proven consistently useful is the assignment of designing a personal coat of arms. Applicants are asked to draw the shape of a shield with six spaces therein and into the spaces to draw a symbol for the answers to the following questions: a) What is your greatest strength or source of strength? b) What would your significant other describe as your greatest strength or source of strength? c) Think of three words which describe you positively and make one symbol. d) What three words would your significant other use to describe you positively? e) What was your greatest fear as a child? f) What is your greatest fear now? During discussion the Director points out the need for caregivers to learn to define and emphasize their positive traits, and to define and deal with their fears. To help patients and families, caregivers must not be dealing with their own identities nor their own fears of dying and grief while in the caregiving role. Hospice provides continuing opportunities for formal and informal personal and professional support for caregivers.

5. *Training.* It is important for applicants to learn about the training process for direct caregivers. Trainees are scheduled to travel with experienced caregivers for as long as individually desirable. This allows a learning experience with direct exposure to selected families in the safe situation of

observer. It is a time for identifying strengths and limitations in order to determine what type of assignment would be appropriate for the individual and therapeutic for the client. The training process takes from two to five months depending on the individual and his or her experience with disease, dying, and grief. This process also allows the opportunity for staff and volunteer to become acquainted in preparation for future personal and professional sharing.

    6. *Knowledge.* It is hospice policy to include trained volunteers in clinical conferences, daily report, and in-service education sessions. Volunteers are encouraged to improve their skills and increase their knowledge in their area of interest through use of the hospice resource center and scheduled meetings with clinical staff. For volunteers who are unable to attend the weekly clinical conference, hospice offers a monthly evening conference with clinical staff present. Volunteers who have been assigned to a case have access to the patient/family record and are kept up to date on the case by the primary nurse. It is effective to have volunteers working as integral team members prepared for making a contribution toward the goals of the patient/family care plan.

    7. *Support.* Volunteers have seven-day-per-week availability of the clinical staff for questions, suggestions, or ventilating. Caregivers are encouraged to talk through personal or work-related problems when they occur, with whatever discipline is most likely to be useful. Volunteers also use each other in this way and become very supportive to each other between scheduled visits and hospice conferences. Volunteers also act as support for staff. Volunteers bring to staff the gift of self, commitment, and caring. Because they are only scheduled between one and three days per week, they bring to full-time staff times of refreshment and renewal. It is not uncommon to see staff socializing with a volunteer at the end of a long, harried day of crises. Volunteers also support staff by taking on innumerable tasks which are essential but for which there are not enough hours in the day to complete, such as errands, filing, xeroxing, resource research, and book reviewing. The most supportive volunteer role is, of course, the responsible way they accomplish their regularly scheduled

assignments. Hospice volunteers can be counted on for quality performance.

8. *Confidentiality.* The public is keenly interested in the details of hospice care. Personnel working with hospice must be especially sensitive to the importance of strict patient/family confidentiality while working with hospice. It is difficult to describe hospice care without using examples. Staff and volunteers who work directly with patients and their families must resist the temptation and maintain a rigid silence about patient and family information, even with their own families and best friends. Patients and families are discussed only with the Home Care Team. A list of Home Care Staff and trained volunteers is given to new trainees.

9. *Active Listening.* The dying and grieving person has the same basic needs as anyone else—for life, safety, and security, for belonging and affection, and for respect and self-respect. Terminal illness turns everyone and everything in a home upside down. The caregiver is often needed in roles which temporarily provide satisfaction for any of the basic needs, not only of the patient, but of the loved ones as well. The most important skill for the volunteer is to know how to listen; to show with the whole self that one is trying to understand what one can do to help. The listening done by caregivers helps people to identify problems and then to communicate those areas where they need help. Hospice knows that communication contains both facts and feelings, and that words frequently express neither. An effective caregiver must learn to listen to words, eyes, body language, family interaction, the environment, and silence.

10. *Active Listening Techniques for Role Playing.* a) Show external signs of listening by eye contact, nodding appropriately, smiling, gestures, posture. b) Ask open-ended questions, "I don't think I understand," or "What do you mean?" c) Be careful that your specific questions are to clarify what the other person wants to communicate, not what you hope he is leading up to. d) Allow time for silence and thought. Calm silence is trust building. e) Observe signals that people want to talk; leaning forward, seeking eye contact with you, stealing glances at you, pursing their lips. Invite them to talk. f) Listen within the

framework of the other person's purpose. Seemingly light social conversation may be leading to a concern or it may also be a need for light social conversation. g) Listen just as intently to the person's nationality, color, religion, experience, conditioning, and feelings as you do to words. h) Use words the speaker himself uses as much as possible. i) Particularly when the person is able to speak only in incomplete ideas, repeat back to him the gist of what he says briefly so he can realize how far he's progressed with the idea, and can continue further if he wants to. j) If words expressing feelings are used, ask a question such as, "You said that made you feel 'alone.' What do you mean?" It is his right to expand or not. k) Don't put words in his mouth. There is a fine line between taking over what he is saying and saying just enough to assist him in putting a complete idea together and sharing it.

POST-COURSE INTERVIEW

The Director of Volunteer Services meets with the applicant to (1) critique the course, (2) mutually evaluate the applicant's suitability for direct patient/family care, (3) formally accept the applicant as a volunteer, and (4) answer questions.

Some applicants have decided during the course that they wish to work in program support instead of direct care tasks. The orientation course gives an understanding of the vital program support provided by backup office work. Also, when the Director is confident that the individual clearly understands the importance of confidentiality, these volunteers may be assigned to the essential work of data collection and record keeping.

Most volunteers who complete the orientation course are mutually assessed to be suitable for direct patient and family care. The Director uses the post-course interview to explain the specialized procedures, policies, and forms which they will be using in their work.

HOME CARE EXPERIENCE

The volunteers who will be working directly with patients and families travel with experienced caregivers into homes for the practical training process. The volunteer keeps a record during this training noting the date, the staff person, and the families visited, so the Director can check the staff person's notes in the patient/family record when questions arise. Staff report the volunteer trainee's progress to the Director, especially when things are going particularly well or particularly poorly. This gives the Director a basis for discussion with the trainee, which is done periodically for the mutual evaluation of the training progress.

The training process is complete when the clinical staff and the trainee agree that the volunteer is ready for assignment. The volunteer understands that he or she will be assigned to a patient or family who needs his/her individual skills and personality. Some volunteers wait for months for their first assignment. During this time, they continue their reading, attend conferences and in-service education sessions, take on in-house projects, and come to hospice community-strengthening social functions.

This method of orientation and training for home care volunteers was developed during the first three years of hospice experience. Faced with the dilemma of patients' and families' need for volunteers and the difficulty of providing supervision for the volunteers while they are alone in homes, hospice concluded that each new caregiver must be well known and thoroughly prepared. The training process requires energy and time, but the result is quality service for patients and families.

PLANNING AND EVALUATION

Volunteers participate in program planning and evaluation. An evaluation of the volunteer program is requested from volunteers annually. The purpose is to give each volunteer an opportunity to make suggestions for the improvement of procedures for orientation, training, communication, and planning. The evaluation is also an opportunity for the volunteer to request a change in position and to express special interests in in-service education programs. Volunteers meet regularly with the Director of Volunteer Services or their immediate supervisor to identify day-to-day problems and suggest changes in departmental procedures.

Each category of service which requires teamwork, in-service education, support, or information updating has been organized into special interest groups which meet regularly for these purposes. For example, the Bereavement Team meets twice each month for in-service education and case discussion, the Reception Team meets monthly for the communication of new information, the nurse volunteers meet monthly to discuss nursing procedures and cases with nursing staff. Each group has a volunteer coordinator who is a member of the Volunteer Advisory Committee. This Committee plans and evaluates the volunteer program with the Director of Volunteer Services. The volunteer leaders also attend all staff meetings as representatives of the volunteer personnel, and staff representatives attend all volunteer meetings. This encourages open communication between staff and volunteers and active volunteer participation in program planning and development.

The Connecticut Hospice has successfully demonstrated that volunteer services can be effectively utilized in an organized program of support for patients with terminal illness and their families. To be effective, volunteers should be utilized as an integral component of hospice care. This incorporates individual personalities, skills, and experiences which will be needed to support the many individual needs of patients and families. The program will change and develop to meet new hospice needs. By sharing in the development of the volunteer program, all hospices share in its growth and strength.

XIII
Regulation and Certification
SUSAN SILVER

Perhaps the most exciting thing about the American Hospice Movement is its grass-roots origin. Across the country, in one community after another, like-minded individuals have come together to discuss and lament the treatment of terminally ill patients in their final days. The hospice alternative emerges as a humanistic ideal, and quite suddenly, health care providers, consumers, and a full range of community professionals and lay people have become the nucleus of a local hospice effort. More than two hundred such groups exist around the country today and the enthusiasm, even desperation, with which they pursue their goal confirms that hospice is an idea whose time has come. However, more than dedication and spirit are needed to make hospice a reality. There comes a time in each community's experience when the gleam in the eye must meet the cold stare of the government and begin to conform to the many requirements imposed by local and federal authorities.

Normally, the transition from informal to formal hospice organization comes with incorporation. In Washington, D.C., for example, a group of concerned individuals met as a committee of the Episcopal Church to assess the need for a hospice in their community. After a year's study they found that a hospice was, indeed, needed but that the Episcopal base was too narrow to reach the entire heterogeneous population that might need care. Consequently, the Episcopal Committee dis-

Susan Silver is Executive Director of the Washington Hospice Society, Inc. in Washington, D.C.

banded in favor of a multi-disciplinary, multi-denominational organization that became incorporated as the Washington Hospice Society, Inc.

The vast majority of hospice organizations are incorporated as not-for-profit entities, although some for-profit or "proprietary" hospices do exist. In either case, articles of incorporation are filed with state officials by an attorney, indicating the nature and purpose of the organization. The organizational structure is expressed in by-laws, also submitted to the state when applying for incorporation. By-laws become the standards of operation and delineate the number and powers of the Board of Directors and specifications for officers, membership, meetings, and the like.

Among non-profit organizations, incorporation is merely the preliminary step to the all-important application for tax-exempt status. Volunteer citizen organizations are frequently effective and productive, but rarely can they flourish effectively without some outside source of funds. At the point at which out-of-pocket expenses become an imposition on volunteers—not to mention the stage at which telephones, office space, or clerical help become necessities—most organizations formulate a budget and begin seeking money from outside sources. Tax-exempt status is essential then (for attracting funds from private philanthropists) since it not only excludes the hospice organization from payment of taxes, but allows contributors to the organization to take an income tax deduction. The most common tax exemption is under article 501(c)(3) of the Internal Revenue Code and prohibits certain activities, including lobbying and partisan politics. The granting of 501(c)(3) status also confers some degree of credibility and oftentimes a *pro bono publico* image.

The acquisition of tax-exempt status can be a lengthy process. Not untypical was the Washington Hospice Society's experience: a full eight months elapsed between the first effort to assemble data for the application and actual granting of the 501(c)(3). While the tax exemption is pending, the only alternative for hospice organizations seeking donations is an arrangement with another already tax-exempt organization to receive funds on behalf of the hospice group. Variously called a channeling agency, conduit, or fiscal agent, the role of the other organization is to receive contributions earmarked for the hospice, then to dispense them to the hospice while monitoring their use for compliance with 501(c)(3) restrictions. The donor takes a tax deduction on the basis of the fiscal agent's 501(c)(3). The fiscal agent may be a church, an established community organization with interests compatible with hospice, or even organizations that specialize in this function. These "professional" fiscal agents claim to give credibility to the hospice project with potential funders because of their own good reputations. Frequently, they charge a fee. In entering into a relationship with any fiscal agent, the terms of the agreement—how the money will be dispensed, how it will be monitored, and fees, if any—must be spelled out in advance. Debate about the use of fiscal agents is ongoing. While some liken it to "laundering" money, others feel that a good fiscal agent can be helpful in putting an organization in a position to solicit funds ahead of the receipt of its own 501(c)(3) status. Hospice, Inc. of New Haven, Connecticut has functioned in a fiscal agent capacity on a non-fee basis for the National Hospice Organization.

Beyond the incorporation and tax exemption stages, state regulations governing hospice organizations diverge quite radically. The new hospice concept has yet to be incorporated into prevailing regulatory and licensing guidelines, and those aspects under state jurisdiction are apt to vary from one state to the next. The uncertainty lies in establishing just what a hospice is. Few states recognize hospice *qua* hospice; most force hospices into other categories. Hospices around the country are variously pegged as home health agencies, skilled nursing facilities, chronic care institutions, general hospitals, and other such labels. Such misplacement of hospice within the health care system too often leads to difficulty in assessment as well as misunderstanding among other pre-existing health care services.

Perhaps the most complex of regulatory processes to which hospice organizations are subject is the comprehensive health planning/certificate of need requirement. Under P.L. 93-641 of 1974—the "Comprehensive Health Planning and

Resources Development Act"—every state and locale must review the necessity of additions to the health care delivery system. Both capital expenditures and new services are subject to scrutiny; thus hospice home care, inpatient care, and expenditures to create a facility are all areas for consideration.

P.L. 93-641 charges the states with reducing health expenditures by eliminating unnecessary or duplicative services. State Health Planning and Development Agencies (SHPDAs) must assess the health care needs of their own state's populations and, with the advice of the State Health Coordinating Council (SHCC), draw up a plan to include all permissible health services for the state. While the SHPDA is a paid staff of health planners, the SHCC is an appointed body comprised of at least 51 percent health care consumers.

Theoretically, then, every health care provider must document the need for the new service he intends to offer and demonstrate to both the SHPDA and the SHCC that it conforms to the state plan. If the provider successfully proves the necessity of his service, it is granted a certificate of need and permitted to proceed as planned.

In actuality, however, many states are far from complete in establishing this comprehensive health planning system. Washington, D.C., for example (which functions in this instance as a state), has no state plan. The SHPDA is not yet fully staffed, nor has the SHCC reached its full quota of members. Consequently, the newness of the planning system, coupled with the newness of the hospice concept, poses a challenge to both sides in trying to incorporate hospice into the health care mainstream.

Generally, the application for a certificate of need addresses the new health services from the points of view of cost, need, accessibility, acceptance, and impact upon similar services. Certainly each of these is an area of concern to hospice planners. Yet, interaction with a panel of the uninitiated is frequently fraught with difficulty for hospice planners, who are rarely called upon to verify their impressionistic evidence within their own hospice circles.

The cost issue is one that can only be determined over time. As existing hospices develop longer records and special hospice demonstration projects generate increased data, cost estimates will become more precise. In the meantime, though, the hospice certificate of need applicant might project cost on the basis of other skilled-nursing home care agencies, prevailing doctors' fees, and comparable services representing components of hospice care. The oft-repeated Hospice, Inc. statistic of a $1,000 total for care in the final three months of life is compelling, but not necessarily transferable to other locations.

But beyond the problem of predicting cost for a service never delivered in a particular community is the difficulty of conveying the pervasive volunteerism and bare-bones budget that so often characterize the fledgling hospice. The typical SHPDA and SHCC are accustomed to reviewing high-budget ventures and, in spite of their mandate to minimize health care expenditures, may regard the relatively economical hospice program with some skepticism. The Washington Hospice Society encountered just such incredulity when a SHCC member asked why no fee was indicated for home care visits by hospice volunteers. The answer, that there would be no charge for volunteer visits, had apparently never occurred to the state appointee. A very careful delineation within the certificate of need application of the hospice's volunteer roots and spirit might lay the groundwork for a proper reading of its budget by state officials.

The questions of need, accessibility, and acceptance are closely interrelated and of particular interest to the consumer-dominated SHCC. Again, however, the conventional wisdom that a person would prefer to die amid familiar and humane caregivers than in isolation in a hospital may not be sufficient for the certificate of need. Individual professionals, hospital discharge planners, and other social service providers may willingly vouch for the need for hospice care based on cases in their own experiences. PSRO-disqualified or inappropriate hospital stays, particularly among cancer patients, may offer strong evidence of the need for alternatives. And generally rising cancer mortality, coupled with a growing demand on home care services for chronic—not terminal—care, demonstrate the widening gap between supply and demand. How-

ever, all of these indications lead only to the conclusion that
present care is inadequate. That hospice could fill the gap
were it available, is another point of which the health planning panel may need to be convinced.

Accessibility, in the case of home care, is easily resolved
in some settings since the home care team visits the patient
wherever he or she is located. As long as travel time is feasible,
all patients can expect to have equal access to care. But, like
acceptance, the issue of access may have political and social
implications to which SHCC consumer members are especially sensitive. Most urban populations are characterized by
substantial portions that are consistently medically under-
served. Factors such as the physical safety of the home care
team, language barriers, and the racial makeup of the team
will determine the willingness to provide care throughout the
city and willingness to accept it. Ability to pay as a criterion
for hospice admission is another fundamental question bearing on accessibility which the certificate of need application
will have to address.

The impact of a hospice program upon similar services
is perhaps the key to determining duplication of service. If
other hospices exist in the applicant's community, a rather
clear-cut question arises of the necessity for an additional program. Far trickier is an explanation of the need for a hospice
facility in a community full of surplus hospital beds or for
hospice home care in an area replete with skilled-nursing
home care agencies. As a matter of policy, both hospitals and
nursing services may oppose the hospice applicant's entry into
the field. Each has the right to submit written or verbal tes-
timony before the SHPDA and SHCC. Either may claim that
the existence of a hospice merely duplicates the services they
offer and would lead to further surpluses and, ultimately, higher
costs to consumers. In more than one state, opponents have
successfully blocked the hospice's attempt to secure a certificate of need and these denials were reversed on appeal only
after planning authorities were convinced of the clear distinc-
tion between hospice care and other home nursing or
hospitalization.

The certificate of need process, from submission of the

application to approval or denial, may take three months. At several junctures the applicant may be called upon for presentation and questioning and to respond to the claims of opponents. Overcoming unfamiliarity with the hospice concept on the part of state authorities is undeniably the greatest obstacle, but once accomplished, the hospice organization is free to bring its plans to fruition.

Any hospice that intends to hire a staff of professional caregivers will undoubtedly want to be reimbursed for services they provide. Patients' payments from their own resources are, of course, one means. But, more likely, patients will depend on insurance to pay their bills. Again, unfamiliarity with hospice creates an obstacle. Currently, private insurance carriers are beginning to investigate hospice, but their progress has been quite slow. Individual hospice groups can negotiate directly with insurance companies heavily represented in their communities to establish a contract for reimbursement. Blue Cross in Washington, D.C., for example, covers hospice care in a small inpatient unit within a nursing home as part of a project to demonstrate quality and cost of care. The same Blue Cross has indicated a willingness to work an arrangement for coverage of home care with the Washington Hospice Society.

In general, negotiations with private carriers may proceed more easily as each sees the others falling in line. However, hospice is apparently still far from enjoying full coverage for its comprehensive program of care. Treatment of the whole family, and particularly bereavement follow-up, is not traditionally regarded as part of medical care, and thus is not included for insurance reimbursement. Re-education at both the local and national levels will be essential to broadening perceptions and coverage of hospice care.

In the public sector, Medicare and Medicaid are the backbones of reimbursement for medical services. While Medicare is federally administered and Medicaid is run by the states, there are similar qualifying procedures for health care providers intending to collect payment from these sources.

Lengthy application forms ask details of staffing, policies, and procedures. A home health agency, for instance, is required to offer skilled nursing, physical and occupational therapy, and home health aide services. The licensee must demonstrate the credentials and availability of these professionals as well as supervising mechanisms for coordinating the total program. Acceptance of patients, plan of treatment, and medical supervision must also be delineated. If all criteria are satisfactorily met, a reimbursement rate is set and the hospice is licensed to bill Medicare and Medicaid directly for the services it renders to patients eligible under these programs. Again, however, reimbursement is restricted as to number of visits and type of care offered.

One could hardly overlook the recurring theme in hospice development: hospice does not quite fit the system. Its emphasis on a multi-disciplinary team of caregivers—some of whom have never before been considered part of a medical team, and on care of the entire family, especially during bereavement—challenges us to rethink our definitions of medical care. Individually, Americans are becoming enthusiastic about hospice, and gradually the state and federal governments are embracing it as well. Several states have adopted legislation setting apart hospice in a category of its own within the health care system. The effect will be the alleviation of restrictions and requirements more appropriate to curative nursing services.

The federal government has entered the hospice field, first by arrangement with individual hospices to provide services to cancer patients under contracts with the National Cancer Institute. More recently, a series of demonstration projects are being designated for whom Medicare and Medicaid restrictions will be waived, and the full range of hospice services will be reimbursable. These projects will generate the all-important data on hospice cost-effectiveness that traditional third-party payors await before committing themselves to coverage for hospice care. If the statistics prove favorable, as hospice planners anticipate, we can expect a more rapid integration of hospice all along the system, from certificate of need to insurance reimbursement.

Bibliography*

Adams, James R. *The Sting of Death: A Leader's Guide for a Study Course on Death and Bereavement.* New York: Seabury Press, 1974.

Adelman, S. E. "Dying Patient: An unspoken dialogue." *New Physician* 20 (1971): 706-708.

Aging Magazine, December 1978. Special section on coming to terms with death.

Aldwinckle, Russell. *Death in the Secular City: Life After Death in Contemporary Theology and Philosophy.* Grand Rapids: Eerdmans Publishing Company, 1972.

Alsofrom, Judy. "The Hospice Way of Dying." *American Medical News,* 21 February 1977: 7-9.

Alsop, Stewart. *Stay of Execution.* Philadelphia: Lippincott, 1973.

Aries, Philippe. *Western Attitudes Toward Death From the Middle Ages to the Present.* Baltimore: Johns Hopkins Press, 1974.

Aring, Charles. *The Understanding Physician.* Detroit: Wayne University Press, 1971.

Ashley, Beth. "Death Without Pain: A Dying Man Tells How Hospice Helps." Reprint. *Independent Journal,* 15 November 1976.

Baqui, Mufti Abdul, and Joseph, Rabbi B. "Jewish and Muslim Teaching Concerning Death: A St. Joseph's Hospice Occasional Paper." London: St. Joseph's Hospice.

Barber, Bernard. "Compassion in Medicine: Toward New Definitions and New Institutions." *New England Journal of Medicine* 295 (October 2, 1976): 939-943.

Bare, J. Donald, *et al.,* eds. *Death and Ministry: Pastoral Care of the Dying and the Bereaved.* New York: Seabury Press, 1975.

Barnard, C. N. "Good Death at St. Christopher's Hospice." *Family Health,* April 1973, pp. 40ff.

This bibliography is based on the excellent one in The Hospice Movement *by Sandol Stoddard, published by Stein and Day and reprinted by permission.*

Barrell, L. M. "Crisis Intervention: Partnership in Problem Solving." *Nursing Clinics of North America* 9 (1974): 5-14.

Bartlett, Linda, and Hodgson, Bryan. "Love, the Final Act of Life." *Washington Post,* 24 April 1977.

Becker, Earnest. *The Denial of Death.* New York: Free Press, 1973.

Bluebond-Langner, Myra. *The Private Worlds of Dying Children.* Princeton: Princeton University Press, 1978.

Buckingham, Robert, *et al. The Hospice Concept.* New York: Highly Specialized Promotions, 1977.

Buckingham, R. W., *et al.* "Living with the Dying: Use of the Technique of Participant Observation." *Canadian Medical Association Journal* 115 (1976): 1211-1215.

Bunch, B., and Zahra, D. "Dealing with Death: The Unlearned Role." *American Journal of Nursing* 76 (1976): 1486-1488.

Caldwell, D., and Mishara, B. L. "Research on Attitudes of Medical Doctors Toward the Dying Patient: A Methodological Problem." *Omega* 3 (1972): 341-346.

Chan, Lo-Yi. "Hospice: A New Building Type to Comfort the Dying." Reprint. *AIA Journal,* December 1976.

Charles, Eleanor. "A Hospice for the Terminally Ill." *New York Times,* 13 March 1977.

Choron, Jacques. *Death and Western Thought.* New York: Collier, 1963.

Colen, B. D. "Nurse's Specialty: Care for the Dying." *Washington Post,* 24 August 1975.

Cook, Sarah Sheets, *et al. Children and Dying: An Exploration and Selective Bibliographies.* New York: Health Sciences Publishing Corporation, 1974.

Craig, Y. "Care of the Dying Child." *Nursing Mirror* 137 (1973): 14-16.

Craven, Joan, and Wald, Florence. "Hospice Care for Dying Patients." *American Journal of Nursing* 75 (1975): 1816-1822.

Creighton, S. A., M.D. "The Hospice—Understanding Care for the Terminally Ill." *The Bulletin,* King County Medical Society, October 1975.

Davison, Glen W., ed. *The Hospice: Development and Administration.* Washington, D.C.: Hemisphere Publishing Corporation, 1978.

————. "The Waiting Vulture Syndrome." *Bereavement: Its Psychosocial Aspects.* Edited by B. Schoenberg, *et al.* New York: Columbia University Press, 1975.

————. *Living with the Dying.* Minneapolis: Augsburg, 1975.

Death Education. Special issue on the hospice, 2: 1-2 (Spring/Summer 1978), 230. Washington, D.C.: Hemisphere Publishing Corporation.

Dobihal, Edward F. "Talk or Terminal Care?" *Connecticut Medicine,* 38 (July 1974): 364-367.

————; Lack, S.; Rezendes, D.; and Wald, F. "Principles of Hospice Care." New Haven: Hospice, Inc., 19 February 1975.

Downie, P. A. "Psychotherapy and the Care of the Progressively Ill Patient." *Nursing Times* 69 (1973): 892-893.

————. "Havens of Peace: Hostels for Terminal Patients." *Nursing Times* 69 (16 August 1973), 1068-1070.

Dunphy, J. Englebert. "On Caring for the Patient With Cancer." *New England Journal of Medicine*, 295 (5 August 1976): 313-319.

Feifel, Herman. "Death and Dying in Modern America." *Death Education* 1 (1977): 5-14.

————, ed. *The Meaning of Death.* New York: McGraw-Hill, 1969.

Ferris, Theodore P. *Death and Transfiguration.* Maxi Books, Cincinnati: Forward Movement Publications, 1974.

"Filling the Gap Between Home and Hospital: St. Ann's Hospice, England." *Nursing Mirror,* 134: 17 (4 February 1972).

Formby, John, Fr.; Hickey, Rev. Michael; and Jones, Rev. Gordon. "Christian Teaching Concerning Death: A St. Joseph's Hospice Occasional Paper." London: St. Joseph's Hospice.

"For the Terminally Ill, A Hospital That Cares: St. Christopher's Hospice, London." *Medical World News* 15 (19 July 1974): 46-47.

Found, K. I. "Dealing with Death and Dying Through Family-Centered Care." *American Journal of Nursing* 7 (1977): 53-64.

Fox, S. "Death of a Child." *Nursing Times* 68 (1972): 1322-1323.

Frase, Arthur. *Living Through Grief and Growing with It.* New York: Harper and Row, 1977.

Friehofer, P., *et al.* "Nursing Behaviors in Bereavement: An Exploratory Study." *Nursing Research* 25 (1976): 332-337.

Galton, V. A. "Cancer Nursing at St. Christopher's Hospice." *Proceedings of the National Conference on Cancer Nursing.* Chicago: American Cancer Society, 1973.

Garner, Jim. "Palliative Care: It's the Quality of Life Remaining That Matters." *CMA Journal* 115 (17 July 1976): 179-180.

Gatch, Milton McC. *Death, Meaning and Mortality in Christian Thought and Contemporary Culture.* New York: Seabury Press, 1969.

Glaser, Barney G., and Strauss, Anselm L. *Awareness of Dying.* Chicago: Aldine, 1965.

Goleman, Daniel. "We are Breaking the Silence About Death." *Psychology Today,* September 1976, pp. 44f.

Grollman, Earl A., ed. *Concerning Death: A Practical Guide for the Living.* Boston: Beacon Press, 1974.

Harker, B. L. "Cancer and Communications Problems: A Personal Experience." *Psychiatry in Medicine* 3 (1972): 163-171.

Hendin, David. *Death as a Fact of Life.* New York: Norton, 1973.

Hines, William. "An Easier Way of Death for Victims of Cancer." *Chicago Sun-Times,* 29 August 1975, p. B7.

"Home Care of the Cancer Patient." *Proceedings of the American Cancer Society Conference.* Syracuse, N.Y., May 10, 1973.

"Hospice for the Dying Planned in Greater New Haven." *Hospital Management* 112 (August 1973): 19.

"Hospice: Pilot Project." Pamphlet. New York: St. Luke's Hospital Center.

"Hospice." *Thanatos,* March 1977, pp. 6-11.

Ingles, Thelma. "St. Christopher's Hospice." *Nursing Outlook* 22 (December 1974): 759-763.

Jaffe, L., and Jaffe, A. "Terminal Cancer and the Coda Syndrome." *American Journal of Nursing* 75 (1976): 1938-1940.

Jung, C. G. *Memories, Dreams, Reflections.* New York: Random House, 1965.

Kastenbaum, R. "Toward Standards of Care for the Terminally Ill: That a Need Exists." *Omega,* 6: 2 (1975), 77.

Kerstein, M. D. "Care for the Terminally Ill: A Hospice." *American Journal of Psychiatry* 129 (August 1972): 237-238.

Kobrzycki, P. "Dying with Dignity at Home." *American Journal of Nursing* 75 (1975): 312-313.

Krant, M. J. *Dying and Dignity: The Meaning and Control of a Personal Death.* Springfield: Charles C. Thomas, 1974.

Kron, Joan. "Designing a Better Place to Die." *New York Magazine,* 1 March 1976, pp. 43-49.

————. "Learning to Live With Death." *Philadelphia Magazine,* April 1973, pp. 82f.

————. "The Good News About the Bad News." *New York Magazine,* 21 July 1975.

Kübler-Ross, Elisabeth, *Death. The Final Stage of Growth.* Englewood Cliffs: Prentice-Hall, 1975.

————. *On Death and Dying.* New York: Macmillan, 1969.

————. *Questions and Answers on Death and Dying.* New York: Macmillan, 1974.

Lack, Sylvia. "Philosophy and Organization of a Hospice Program." Pamphlet. New Haven: Hospice, Inc.

Lamerton, Richard. "Euthanasia." Reprint. *Nursing Times,* 21 February 1974.

————. "The Need for Hospices." *Nursing Times* 71 (23 January 1975): 155-157.

————. "Vegetables?" Reprint. *Nursing Times,* 1 August 1974.

Lamerton, Richard, and Lack, Sylvia, eds. *The Hour of Our Death.* London: Macmillan, 1974.

LeShan, Eda. *Learning to Say Good-By: When a Parent Dies.* New York: Macmillan Publishing Company, 1976.

LeShan, L. "The World of the Patient in Severe Pain of Long Duration." *Journal of Chronic Diseases* 17 (1964): 119-126.

Levinson, P. "Obstacles in the Treatment of Dying Patients." *American Journal of Psychiatry* 132 (1975): 28-32.

Lewis, C. S. *A Grief Observed.* New York: Seabury Press, 1961.

————. *The Problem of Pain.* London: The Centenary Press, 1940.

Lewis, Tony. "Hospice Gave Them an Alternative." Reprint. *Twin Cities Times.* Corte Madera, California, 30 March 1977.

————. "Hospice of Marin: Caring for the Terminally Ill at Home." Reprint. *Twin Cities Times.* Corte Madera, California, 30 March 1977.

Liegner, L. M. "St. Christopher's Hospice, 1974. Care of the Dying Patient." *Journal of the American Medical Association* 234 (1975): 1047-1048.

Libman, Joan. "Death's Door: Hospice Movement Stresses Family Care." *The Wall Street Journal,* 27 March 1978.

Mann, S. A. "Coping With a Child's Fatal Illness: A Parent's Dilemma." *Nursing Clinics of North America* 9 (1974): 81-87.

Mannes, Marya. *Last Rights.* New York: Wm. Morrow, 1972.

Martinson, I. M., *et al.* "Home Care for the Child." *American Journal of Nursing* 77 (1977): 1815-1817.

McNulty, Barbara. "St. Christopher's Out-Patients." *American Journal of Nursing,* December 1971, pp. 2328-2330.

Miller, Jack S. *The Healing Power of Grief.* Crossroad Books. New York: Seabury Press, 1978.

Moody, Raymond A., Jr. *Life After Life.* Atlanta: Mockingbird Books, 1975.

Mount, Balfour M.; Jones, Allan; and Patterson, Andrew. "Death and Dying: Attitudes in a General Hospital." *Urology* IV: 6 (December 1974), 741-747.

————; Ajemian, I.; and Scott, J. F. "Use of the Brompton Mixture in Treating the Chronic Pain of Malignant Disease." *CMA Journal,* 17 July 1976, pp. 122-128.

————. "The Problems of Caring for the Dying in a General Hospital." *CMA Journal,* 17 July 1976, pp. 119-124.

Neale, Robert E. *The Art of Dying.* New York: Harper and Row, 1973.

Netsky, Martin D. "Dying in a System of 'Good Care': Case Report and Analysis." *PHAROS,* April 1976, pp. 57-61.

"New Haven Hospice Provides Home Care for the Terminally Ill." Reprint. *American Journal of Nursing,* 74 (April 1974): 717.

Nolan, T. "Ritual and Therapy." *Anticipatory Grief.* Edited by B. Schoenberg, *et al.* New York: Columbia University Press, 1974, pp. 358-364.

Nouwen, Henri. *Reaching Out.* New York: Doubleday, 1975.

————. *The Wounded Healer.* New York: Doubleday, 1972.

————. *With Open Hands.* Notre Dame: Ave Maria Press, 1972.

Noyse, R., and Clancy, J. "The Dying Role: Its Relevance to Improved Patient Care." *Psychiatry* 40 (1977): 41-47.

"On Dying at Home." *Emergency Medicine,* February 1977, pp. 137-141.

"On Dying Well: An Anglican Contribution to the Debate on Euthanasia." Pamphlet. London: Yelf Bros., 1975.

"Optimum Care for Hopelessly Ill Patients." *New England Journal of Medicine* 295 (12 August 1976): 362-364.

Osler, Sir William. *The Student Life and Other Essays.* Boston: Houghton Mifflin, 1931.

Paige, R. L., and Looney, J. F. "Hospice Care for the Adult." *American Journal of Nursing* 77 (1977): 1812-1815.

"Pain and Suffering—A Special Supplement." *American Journal of Nursing* 74 (1974): 491-520.

"Palliative Care Service: Pilot Project." Montreal: Royal Victoria Hospital, McGill University, 1976.

Parkes, Colin Murray. *Bereavement: Studies of Grief in Adult Life.* Middlesex: Penguin, 1975.

Pellman, D. R. "Learning to Live with Dying." *The New York Times Magazine,* 5 December 1976.

Powledge, Tabitha M. "Death as an Acceptable Subject." *New York Times,* 25 July 1976.

Proulx, J. R. "Ministering to the Dying: A Joint Pastoral and Nursing Effort." *Hospital Progress* 56 (1975): 62-63.

Quint, Jeanne. *The Nurse and the Dying Patient.* New York: Macmillan, 1967.

Rahner, Karl. *On the Theology of Death.* Crossroad Books. New York: Seabury, 1976.

Reeves, Robert B., Jr., *et al.,* eds. *Pastoral Care of the Dying and the Bereaved: Selected Readings.* New York: Health Sciences Publishing Corporation, 1973.

Rhein, Reginald W., Jr. "The Health Cost 'Crisis.' " *Medical World News,* 21 February 1977, pp. 57-72.

Richardson, J. "On Dying and Dying Well." *Proceedings of the Royal Society of Medicine* 70 (1977): 71-73.

Rossman, Parker. "A Prophetic Ministry to the Dying." Interview with Edward F. Dobihal. *The Christian Century,* 21 April 1976, pp. 384-387.

Ryder, Claire F., and Ross, Diane M. "Terminal Care: Issues and Alternatives." *Public Health Reports,* January/February 1977, pp. 20-29.

Saunders, Cicely. "And From Sudden Death. . . ." Reprint. *Frontier,* Winter 1961.

————. "Care of the Dying." *A Nursing Times Publication.* 2nd ed. London, 1976.

————. *Care of the Dying.* London: Macmillan, 1959.

_____. "Essentials for a Hospice." Privately printed by St. Christopher's Hospice, London, 1976.

_____. "I Was Sick And You Visited Me." *In the Service of Medicine: A Quarterly Paper*, 42: 2 (July 1965).

_____. "Telling Patients." Reprint. *District Nursing*, September 1965.

_____. "Terminal Care." *Medical Oncology*. Edited by K. D. Bagshawe. Oxford: Blackwell Scientific Publications, 1973.

_____. "The Challenge of Terminal Care." *Scientific Foundations of Oncology*. Edited by T. Symington and R. L. Carter. London: Heinemann, 1975.

_____. "The Last Stages of Life." *American Journal of Nursing*, March 1965, pp. 70-75.

_____. "The Management of Fatal Illness in Childhood." *Proceedings of the Royal Society of Medicine*, 62: 6 (June 1969), 550-553.

_____. "The Management of Terminal Illness." Reprint. Hospital Publications, Ltd., London, 1967.

_____. "The Need for Inpatient Care for the Patient with Terminal Cancer." Anniversary Volume. *Middlesex Hospital Journal*, 72: 3 (February 1973).

_____. "The Symptomatic Treatment of Incurable Malignant Disease." *Prescriber's Journal*, October 1964, pp. 68-73.

_____. "Training for the Practice of Clinical Gerontology: The Role of Social Medicine." *Interdisciplinary Topics of Gerontology* 5 (1970): 72-78.

_____. "Treatment of Intractable Pain in Terminal Cancer." *Proceedings of the Royal Society of Medicine*, 56: 191.

_____. "Watch With Me." Reprint. *Nursing Times*, 26 November 1965.

_____, ed. *The Management of Terminal Malignant Disease*. London: Edward Arnold, 1977.

Schneidman, E. S., ed. "Death Work and Stages of Dying." *Death, Current Perspectives*. Palo Alto: Mayfield, 1976, pp. 443-451.

Shephard, David A. E. "Principles and Practice of Palliative Care." *CMA Journal*, 5 March 1977, pp. 522-526.

_____. "Terminal Care: Towards an Ideal." *CMA Journal*, 17 July 1976, pp. 97-98.

Shimkin, M. B. "Implementation of the Hospice Concept." In *Science and Cancer*, DHEW (NIH) 15-568, 1973.

Shinn, Roger L. *Life, Death and Destiny*. Miniature Books. Cincinnati: Forward Movement Publications, 1971.

"Standards of Care for the Terminally Ill." *Ars Moriendi Convention Report*. Columbia, Maryland, November 1974.

Steinberg, Marion. "Death With Dignity." *The Journal of the Connecticut Business and Industry Association*, 54: 11 (November 1976).

Steinfels, Peter, and Veatch, Robert M., eds. *The Hastings Center*

Report: Death Inside Out. New York: Harper, 1974.

Stoddard, Sandol. *The Hospice Movement.* New York: Stein and Day, 1978.

Strauss, Anselm L. "Problems of Death and the Dying Patient." *Aging in Modern Society.* Edited by Alexander Simon and Leon J. Epstein. Washington: American Psychiatric Association, 1968.

Taylor, Michael J., ed. *The Mystery of Suffering and Death.* Staten Island, New York: Alba House, 1973.

Tolstoi, L. *The Death of Ivan Ilych.* New York: Health Sciences Publishing Corporation, 1973.

Tozer, Eliot. "Hospices." *Practical Psychology for Physicians,* September 1976, pp. 61-67.

Troup, Stanley B., and Greene, William A., eds. *The Patient, Death and the Family.* New York: Scribner, 1974.

Twycross, R. G. "Choice of Strong Analgesic in Terminal Cancer: Diamorphine or Morphine?" *Pain* (The Journal of the International Association for the Study of Pain), 3: 2 (April 1977): 93-104.

_____. "Clinical Experience With Diamorphine in Advanced Malignant Disease." Reprint. *International Journal of Clinical Pharmacology,* 9: 184.

_____. "Diseases of the Central Nervous System: Relief of Terminal Pain." Reprint. *British Medical Journal,* 25 October 1975.

_____. "Principles and Practice of the Relief of Pain in Terminal Cancer." Reprint. *Update,* July 1972.

_____. "Stumbling Blocks in the Study of Diamorphine." *Postgraduate Medical Journal,* May 1973, pp. 309-313.

_____. "The Dying Patient." Pamphlet. London: CMF Publications, 1975.

_____. "The Terminal Care of Patients With Lung Cancer." *Postgraduate Medical Journal,* October 1973, pp. 732-737.

Vachon, M. L. S.; Lyall, W. A. L.; and Freeman, S. J. J. "Measurement and Management of Stress in Health Professionals Working with Advanced Cancer Patients." *Death Education* 1 (1978): 365-375.

Veatch, Robert M. *Death, Dying and the Biological Revolution: Our Last Quest for Responsibility.* New Haven: Yale University Press, 1976.

Wald, Florence S. "For Everything There is a Season and a Time to Every Purpose." *The New Physician,* April 1969, pp. 278-285.

Ward, A. M. W. "Impact of a Special Unit for Terminal Care." *Social Science and Medicine* 10 (1976): 373-376.

Wentzel, K. B. "Dying Are the Living: St. Christopher's Hospice, London." *American Journal of Nursing* 76 (January 1976): 956-957.

Wessel, Morris A. "To Comfort Always." *Yale Alumni Magazine,* June 1972, pp. 17-19.

West, Thomas S. "Approach To Death." Reprint. *Nursing Mirror,*

10 October 1974.

————. "The Final Voyage." *Frontier*, 17: 4 (Winter 1974).

Witzel, L. "Behavior of the Dying Patient." *British Medical Journal* 2 (1975): 81-82.

Woodward, Kenneth L. "There Is Life After Death." Interview with Dr. Elisabeth Kübler-Ross. *McCall's*, August 1976, pp. 97ff.

Yalom, I. D. "Group Therapy with the Terminally Ill." *American Journal of Psychiatry* 23 (1977): 20-24.

Yates, Susan. "Experience With Dying Patients." *American Journal of Nursing*, 73: 6 (June 1973).

Xiques, Linda. "Dying At Home." Reprint. *Pacific Sun*, 28 January 1977.

Zorza, Rosemary and Victor. "The Death of a Daughter." *The Washington Post*, 22 January 1978.

NOTE: For further reference, the editors also recommend *The Thanatology Library*, a comprehensive (over 250 titles) annotated catalogue of "books and audio visual materials on Death, Bereavement, Loss, and Grief." It is available from:

Highly Specialized Promotions
228 Clinton Street
Brooklyn, New York 11201

Slides and Films

HOSPICE: CARE FOR THE LIVING AND DYING. *National Council of Churches*, TV Film Library, Room 860, 475 Riverside Drive, New York, N.Y. 10027. (212) 870-2575.
30 min. black and white, $12, order number: NC 616.

A proposed hospice in the United States, modeled after St. Christopher's in London, is now being built in New Haven. While the building is going on, services to the terminally ill are taking place, and the Rev. Edward Dobihal (President of Hospice, Inc.) and Dr. Sylvia Lack (Medical Director) discuss with Herb Kaplow creative ways of dealing medically and spiritually with the terminally ill and their families.

HOW COULD I NOT BE AMONG YOU? *Thomas Reichman,* Benchmark Films, 145 Scarboro Rd., Briarcliff Manor, N.Y. 10510.
30 min. color, 1970.

Tom Reichman has made a visual accompaniment for the writings of poet Ted Rosenthal, who at 30 learned he had leukemia. In free verse and awkward prose, Rosenthal expresses his reactions and shares his philosophy. There is much to absorb and the film can be viewed with profit more than once. The film is a song of dying. Its message is to live and love while you can.

Rosenthal responds to his prognosis with an intensified appreciation of the people and places around him. The terminal diagnosis releases him from previous cares. He feels free and unafraid. As his illness proceeds he describes his symptoms stoically but finally admits that he is "sick of dying" and that it is a "waste of time."

The film is well done; it is artistic and aesthetic. The language of the poet is emotional and "gutsy" enough to perhaps offend some viewers. After all, he was not working with a pleasant subject.

DEATH. *Arthur Barron,* Filmakers Library, Inc., 290 W. End Avenue, New York, N.Y. 10023.
40 min. black and white, 1968

This film is a documentary originally produced for NET in 1968 and is still a useful record. The staff of Calvary Hospital in the Bronx, New York, presents the problem of caring for the dying cancer patient.

The film opens with a hospital congregation at mass, singing in the chapel. This is the happiest scene in the entire film. In the next scene a physician states that the medical profession does not really know how to handle the terminally ill and as a result such patients tend to get isolated in a hospital—like Calvary—that is willing to take them. There are a number of shots of patients being interviewed by members of the health care teams. All these patients speak of their excruciating pain and look as though they surely feel it.

One doctor kids the patients as he makes his rounds. "All right, everybody up!" "Why don't you people talk to each other in this ward? I think we ought to get rid of that TV."

The staff is shown in a seminar on dying where they discuss their own feelings and experiences with death and grief. In the orientation of new employees, they are told not to plan to cure the patients, but to care for them and make them comfortable. Patients are asked what advice they would give to new employees.

In one vignette a new aide insists that a patient looks all right when he is in pain and emaciated. He finally says, "Yeah, it's a great life." Later, he is shown being pronounced dead, wrapped in sheets and wheeled to the morgue while staff guards the halls to make sure no patients see this.

The last part of the film deals with a fifty-two-year-old single man, Albro Pearsall. He tells his reaction to the care he has been given in the hospital. Albro's brother and sister-in-law share their views of what his life has meant. He complains of memory loss, weakness, pain, and loss of appetite. Home movie clips and snapshots of earlier, healthier times include family get-togethers, Albro in his Coast Guard uniform, and his apartment and keepsakes.

His former employer describes his work as excellent even though he was a loner. Albro describes himself as meticulous and seems to regret time spent in housework instead of outside activities. His employer remarks that "thousands leave no mark." But Mr. Pearsall has left an indelible mark through this movie.

He said, "All I am interested in now is relief from pain." In a visit with the chaplain, Albro says he has asked the Lord to take the pain from his body. His deathbed is also depicted along with his trip to the morgue and the funeral home.

This film honestly portrays dying as it has usually been accomplished by patients everywhere and unfortunately still is in many places. The stark reality of pain, isolation, and desperation that is presented does not produce a pleasant experience for the viewer, but, nevertheless, one in which much can be learned about caring for the dying.

THE DIGNITY OF DEATH. *ABC News,* 1973.

The most noticeable recurring sound in this film about St. Christopher's Hospice in London is, strangely enough since the average patient admitted has one month to live, laughter. In the opening scene with a doctor and nurse at a patient's bedside, the laughter of all three claims one's attention. Then, like an air-filled ball that cannot be kept under water, it keeps bouncing up here and there throughout the film. St. Christopher's Hospice certainly appears to be a happy place.

Children also have an invading presence in the movie. George Watson, the narrator, states, "Visitors are welcome anytime; children are always welcome." St. Christopher's provides a nursery for the staff's children. These children, along with those who visit the patients, make a vital contribution to the atmosphere.

Hospice is a medieval word that meant a stopping place for travelers, according to Cicely Saunders, who founded St. Christopher's in 1967. In this case it is a stopping place for patients, families, and even for staff who sometimes come right out of their professional schools to settle some personal dilemmas about death. St. Christopher's mission is the "spiritual treatment and medical care of dying men and women." Its goal is to "combine the learning of science and the wisdom of religion to relieve physical pain and mental anguish of dying patients and their families."

The physical setting of the hospice is bright and airy. There are wards with each bed having a colorful curtain around it. The patient's personal additions of flowers, paintings, personal articles, and lounge chairs give a feeling of warmth. "An untidy ward is a good ward," says Dr. Saunders in reference to the clutter of the patient's personal belongings. The nurses themselves also add to this atmosphere by wearing aqua uniforms.

The Christian religion also plays an integral part in the activities of St. Christopher's. According to Dr. Saunders, "We have found community but also something beyond ourselves." There are scenes of a chapel service with communion being served, two patients in different interviews mentioning religion, and interviews with both the chaplain, the Reverend Philip Edwards, and the Reverend Ed Dobihal, who has started a hospice in New Haven. The chaplain notes that no religious pressure is put on anyone.

This film presents the hospice concept of caring for the dying patient in a most favorable light. Two significant areas of St. Christopher's barely receive mention, however. The use of diamorphine (heroin) for the relief of pain along with Dr. Saunder's philosophy of drug use (which she calls "polypharmacy") should have been given more attention, along with the bereavement service of the hospice, which follows families for up to 18 months. Nevertheless, the film does provide a rather comprehensive glimpse of St. Christopher's Hospice in less than 30 minutes.

TERMINAL CANCER: The Hospice Approach to Pain Control (Part 1) with *Sylvia A. Lack*, M. D., Medical Director of Hospice, Inc., New Haven, Conn.
19 min. color, videotape, NCME, Roche, 1977.

Of all patients with terminal cancer, 50 percent require analgesics to control pain; 40 percent have pain that is moderate to severe in intensity. Proper attention to the details of prescribing medications will assure that the patient remains both alert and free of pain. Dr. Lack shows the viewer how to do this in the videotape.

Since 1967, when Dr. Cicely Saunders established the first hospice in England, twenty-five more have come into existence in that country. The first hospice was begun in the United States in 1971 at New Haven. There are now approximately forty groups planning hospice programs in this country, and more than ten are already providing patient and family care.

"Pain and cancer are not synonymous," according to the narrator, Dr. Lack. She maintains an opinion based on studies in England that 50 percent of all cancer patients have no pain. She does admit, however, that pain is the dominant symptom associated with cancer. She states further that "terminal cancer pain is purposeless, chronic, generalized, and has no perceivable end."

Dr. Lack strongly recommends administering analgesics before pain recurs. The formula for successful pain control at Hospice, Inc., in New Haven is (1) regular administration, (2) adequate dosage, and (3) oral medication whenever possible. She explains that a psychological dependence occurs only if a patient experiences pain between doses. Many physicians prescribe pain medication "prn" (as needed). Dr. Lack feels that this has no place in caring for terminal patients who, once treatment begins, should never be allowed to feel their pain and thus have to ask for relief. In fact, dosages are normally reduced as patients grow more confident that their pain is being controlled. They also become more relaxed. Excerpts from interviews with three patients are interspersed through the tape to verify Dr. Lack's conclusions. By giving medications orally in cherry syrup, the pain of an injection is avoided. When injected medications are needed, the patient usually requires institutionalization.

"Brompton's mixture," the famous British liquid composed of

heroin, cocaine, alcohol, syrup, and chloroform water is not used in New Haven. It is not needed. Instead they use various ratios of morphine or methadone and phenothiazines.

While this videotape will be most useful to physicians who treat the terminally ill, it is also quite informative for all those in the health care field who work with those dying of cancer. Much more detail about dosages is charted and explained in the videotape than has been attempted here. Yet, Dr. Lack emphasizes the importance that all staff who work around the cancer patient maintain a commitment that pain can and will be controlled. "No patient should want to die because of the pain being suffered."

TERMINAL CANCER: The Hospice Approach to the Family (Part 2) with *Sylvia A. Lack,* M. D., Medical Director of Hospice, Inc., New Haven, Conn.
19 min. color, videotape, NCME, Roche, 1977.

Caring for terminally ill patients and their families is different from most patient care; it's "curiously satisfying," according to Dr. Lack, the narrator of this videotape. Brief segments of interviews with various members of one family by Dr. Lack, a social worker, and a nurse are inserted throughout to give credence to views being asserted.

The approach to families espoused is that taken by Hospice, Inc., which was funded in part by the National Cancer Institute.

The family is seen as the unit of care in terminal illness and is incorporated as part of the health care team. Hospice staff teach the family to care for the patient at home and to provide nursing care until readmission or death. Thus, the family can apply its hard-won knowledge of the patient's particular likes and dislikes. The family may prefer to hire someone to help with household work rather than a nurse if the family gives good nursing care. Patients and their families have available a continuous telephone service provided by the hospice. Families frequently test this at first to be sure it is there, but then their use of it diminishes.

Families are educated to budget their strength and finances with a terminal patient since things will get worse rather than better and easier. Admission to this hospice or a hospital, they are assured, doesn't mean that the family has failed, only that their patient's needs have changed. The hospice encourages families to be involved in the patient's care even during institutionalization. Dr. Lack believes that this reduces their guilt feelings at the time of death. Flexible visiting hours provide easy access to the patient, the presence of children (a sign of one's own mortality), permission to help care for the patient, and space for families such as a family room.

One thing puzzled me about this program. The purpose of the hospice was stated as follows: "to meet the physical, spiritual and emotional needs of patients and their families." Yet, no further word was uttered throughout this tape (or Part I of the series) about meeting the spiritual needs. No chaplain was pictured in any of the scenes. This program should prove to be helpful, informative, and hopefully, mind-changing to physicians and those in administrative positions. Nurses could learn much from it that would make their work easier and more interesting as well as allowing families to feel more useful. Social workers and chaplains should be able to support most of the suggestions.

AUDIOVISUAL NOTES

A Conference on the Dying Child. Barbara Brodie, Carol Alexander, Rosalie Belniak, Barbara Logue, 16 mm, 44 min, black and white, 1967. Presented are the problems of nurses' emotions in caring for the dying child, how they must accept them and the emotions of the family, how the child learns the concept of death, inadvertent changes in the care of the child who is dying, and how support might be given to child and parents alike.

A Special Kind of Care. American Journal of Nursing, 16mm, 13 min, color, 1968. Demonstrates the emotional impact of a diagnosis of advanced cancer on a family.

Basic Principles of Terminal Care. F. R. Gusterson, 28 min. Need for key manager for care of each patient and for communication; relationship with patient and family to gain confidence; control of pain; etc. Audience—GP's, junior hospital staff, nurses, Or. MRSF.

Care of the Patient Who is Dying. Filmstrip, 35 mm, color (cassette/record) with instructor's guide. Trainex Corporation. Guides the learner to accept the events accompanying death in the hospital and to cope with the emotional reactions that occur in the hospital staff, the family, and the patient.

Care of the Patient With Terminal Cancer. Filmstrip, 35 mm, color (cassette/record) with instructor's guide. Trainex Corporation. Focuses on many aspects of physical care and psychological support necessary for patients with terminal cancer.

Group Therapy With a Terminal Patient. Videotape, 50 min. Produced by Walter Reed Army Medical Center, Washington, D.C. WR 109-5, Reel No. 61, 1975. This tape consists of an interview with a terminal patient concerning marital problems associated with a terminal illness and other psychosocial elements of treating the needs of the terminal patient.

Guidelines for Interacting With the Dying Patient. Filmstrip, 35 mm, and 1 cassette, color (1/2-track mono. 22 min), 1972. Concept Media presents perspectives on dying—program 4.

Hazards and Challenges in Providing Care. Filmstrip, color, 35 mm, and 1 cassette (1/2-track mono. 28 min). Concept Media presents perspectives on dying—program 3.

Just a Little Time. Barey-Callaci-Video Nursing, 16 mm, color, 21 min, 1973. Production made possible by a grant from the Samuel S. Fels Fund, Philadelphia, Pa. A documentary exploration of the shared experience of a 49-year-old terminally ill woman and her nurse, Mrs. Dona LeBlanc, a nurse specialist in oncology. The dialogue reveals the unique rewards as well as the special problems involved in the relationship between the nurse and the dying patient.

Just a Little Time. Barey-Callaci-Video Nursing, 1973. This audiocassette and study guide are designed to be used in conjunction with the film of the same title. The recording consists of a conference among nursing staff concerned with developing a plan of care for the patient in the film, a 49-year-old terminally ill woman.

Management of the Terminally Ill: The Family. Network for Continuing Medical Education, VC ¾ in, black and white, 16 min. Offers practical help to physicians in dealing with the dying patient.

Nursing Management of the Dying Patient. American Cancer Society, 5″ reel/cassette, 21 min. Points out the varied ways in which people perceive and react to their dying, and how each needs to be treated as an individual.

Religion and the Clergy. Videorecording, University of Washington Health Sciences Learning Resources Center, 1 cassette, 35 min, black and white, 1974.

Terminal Patients: Their Attitudes and Yours. 16 mm, 16 min, Abbott Laboratories, 1974. Explores staff attitudes toward caring for the terminally ill and probes the thoughts of two dying patients.

Till Death Do Us Part. Videotape, 55 min. Produced by Walter Reed Army Medical Center, Washington, D.C., WR 109-75, Reel No. 61, 1975. The tape depicts psychotherapy interviews with five terminal patients. The emphasis is both content- and process-oriented. This program demonstrates feelings, attitudes, and interpretations of patients undergoing treatment of cancer.

To Take A Hand. Motion picture, University of Texas, M.D. Anderson Hospital and Tumor Institute at Houston, 1 reel, 16 mm, 17 min, color, 1969.